HELP!

First Aid for everyday emergencies

Norman Bezzant

A. G. R. Bone
C.StJ., A E., S.E.N., SE Area Commissioner, London District, St John Ambulance Brigade

E. C. Dawson
M.B., B Sc., C.StJ., London District Surgeon, St John Ambulance Brigade

Catherine Stretton
S.R.N., R.C.N.T., Deputy London District Nursing Officer, St John Ambulance Brigade

Foreword by
Sir Hedley Atkins
K.B.E., D.M., M.Ch., P.P.R.C.S., L.R.C.P.

Collins : Glasgow and London

Published by William Collins Sons and Company Ltd
Glasgow and London

© E. C. Dawson, C. M. Stretton, A. G. R. Bone,
Norman Bezzant 1978

Line drawings by John Harrold
© 1978 William Collins Sons and Company Ltd

ISBN 0 00 435008 1

Printed in Great Britain

Contents

Foreword   6

Introduction   How to use this book   7
                Accident prevention   7
                Equipment   8
                Help routine   8
                Priorities   8
                Shock   9
                Coping with confidence   9

Section I   Being prepared   11

Chapter 1   Accidents—how they happen and
                how to avoid them   12
                How to prevent accidents   14
                Common accidents   14
                Accidents room-by-room   17
                Modern adhesives   20
                Sports and hobbies   20
                On the road   21
                Summary   21

Chapter 2   Equipment   22
                For the home   22
                First aid box in the car   24
                Applying the triangular bandage   25
                Applying compressed dressings   27
                Applying conforming bandages   28

Chapter 3   Taking action   29
                The preliminary routine   29
                The emergency services routine   30
                The examination   31
                The diagnosis   32
                The treatment   33
                The recovery position   34
                The kiss of life routine   34
                Heart massage routine   36
                The coloured casualty   37

	Summary of the help routine	38
	Continuing care	38
	Pulse rate	39
	Shock	40
Section II	Routines for giving assistance	41
Chapter 4	Breathing	42
	The kiss of life routine	43
	The artificial respiration routine	44
	Common causes of failure to breathe	45
	Heart massage (cardiac compression)	46
	Summary of breathing routines	49
Chapter 5	Bleeding	50
	Symptoms of heavy loss of blood	50
	Surface bleeding	51
	Bleeding from within the body	53
	Anti-coagulants	58
Chapter 6	Unconsciousness	59
	Causes of unconsciousness	61
Chapter 7	Burns and scalds	69
	Some important don'ts	70
	General treatment	70
	Circumstances requiring special treatments	72
Chapter 8	Bones and muscles	75
	Diagnosis of fractures	76
	Treatments for special parts	77
	Dislocations	82
	Sprains	83
	Strains	83
Chapter 9	Poisons	84
	Some important don'ts	84
	Common poisons	85
	Poisoning through the skin	86
Chapter 10	Bites and stings	88
	Dog and cat bites	88

	Scratches, especially from cats	89
	Snake bites	89
	Insects and plants	90
	Dangerous marine creatures	91
Chapter 11	Superficial wounds	93
	Two don'ts to remember	93
Section III	Special circumstances	96
Chapter 12	Road accidents	97
	The road accident and you	97
	Arriving on the scene	97
	Deciding to stop at an accident	98
	Organizing the situation	98
	Dealing with the casualties	100
Chapter 13	Holiday and sports injuries	102
	Soccer and rugby	103
	Racket, bat and stick games	103
	Athletics	104
	Water sports	104
	Sports of conveyance	105
	Winter sports	106
	Big game hunting	106
	Climbing and pot-holing	107
	Excessive heat	108
	Conclusion	109
Chapter 14	Accidents related to age groups	110
	Infants—birth to 5 years	110
	Children—5 to 10 years	113
	Young people—10 to 20 years	113
	Adults—20 to 45 years	113
	Adults—45 to 65 years	113
	The elderly aged over 65 years	113
Chapter 15	Emergency childbirth	117
	The preliminary routine	117
	Assessment of the situation	118
	The three stages of labour	118
	The birth routine	120
Index		121

Foreword

When I was invited to write the Foreword to this book I felt very honoured. I have known the authors now for some years and have had experience of their knowledge in First Aid matters, their skills in imparting this knowledge and their complete dedication to the objectives of the St John Ambulance Brigade. Indeed to be associated with them has been an education in itself.

To doctors, nurses, ambulance crews and police, accidents are commonplace. Because of their training these experts know precisely what to do and in what order. Although I have been in surgical practice now for more than forty years I have found that I am still uncertain how to handle an emergency on the few occasions when I have encountered a disaster in the street or in the home. This excellent book tells you exactly what to do in almost every possible emergency.

Readers may, like myself, have had little experience of dealing with the drama of an emergency on the spot as is inevitable if this happens to a member of your own family in the home or even to yourself; or if you are faced with a casualty hit or run over by a car in the street.

Many of us are untrained and, not knowing what to do, our first reaction may be to turn away, not because we are unwilling, but because we are UNABLE to help.

At last we have a book that every housewife, every car driver and every athlete should have at hand so that he or she can act in a sensible, helpful way knowing that the course pursued is in the best interest of the injured, that application of this knowledge may even save life.

Help! gives easy and straightforward instruction in simple everyday language for almost any situation that can arise. To be prepared the reader must do two things:—

First, read Section I of this book.

Second, purchase the relatively small amount of essential equipment recommended.

Then, when an accident happens, you will not be taken unawares but you will remain calm and efficient and know what to do.

Help! has been produced at a price which brings it within the reach of everyone and happily its sales will contribute to the funds of the St John Ambulance Brigade.

I can with the greatest confidence recommend this book to unqualified members of the public.

BE PREPARED. YOU NEVER KNOW.

Sir Hedley Atkins
K.B.E., D.M., M.Ch., P.P.R.C.S., L.R.C.P.

Introduction

How to use this book

This book is to help you cope when accidents happen. For example, when one of the family cuts a hand with a sharp kitchen knife; driving to work, you are first on the scene of a bad road accident; a player in your team injures his leg in a game of football; a child falls off his bicycle, slashing open his arm; a colleague at work injures himself on the machine he is operating. Ask yourself, what could you do about these accidents? This book will give you the confidence to assist and prevent people suffering unnecessarily when no professional aid is available or while you are waiting for it to arrive.

Help! is not intended to be a substitute for your family doctor or qualified first aider, but is to be used as a guide and ready reference in an emergency. It tells you what to do until the professionals come.

In order to be of real assistance when there has been an accident, you must be prepared beforehand. You may be able to do little or nothing, or may even make matters worse by taking action without basic knowledge. Bad handling can often complicate a situation and do irreparable damage. So, be ready for an accident when it happens simply by reading the first Section of *Help!* and by taking the action it suggests in advance. This is how you do it.

Do not wait until an emergency has arisen, but start reading the book first. Learn the simple routine outlined, which we call the Help Routine, and then you will know how to deal with any emergency when it arises.

Accident prevention

Read the first chapter, which deals with this subject. You will see how and why most accidents happen, and how they can often be avoided. Many accidents are the fault of other people. If a builder on a scaffold drops a brick, it may be impossible to prevent it from landing on somebody's head. But the toddler who pulls a saucepan of boiling soup over his face from the front edge of the cooker might have been saved had the soup been heated on one of the back rings, out of his reach.

Equipment

While it is sometimes possible to improvise with materials normally to be found in the home, it is better to have a supply of basic first aid equipment handy, preferably in a metal or plastic box. Sheets have been used since time immemorial for stripping into bandages or substituting for ladders, but most of us would trust other people's lives to them rather than our own. *Help!* specifies the equipment necessary for the home and the car, and suggests the supplies that are always useful in the medicine cupboard.

On the pages following the specification of equipment are the simplest possible instructions, illustrated where necessary, for using it. These instructions contain suggestions for exercises such as bandaging; they are well worth trying before you need to apply the techniques under the pressure of an emergency.

The Help Routine

The next Chapter of *Help!* tells you how to handle an accident. Although you will not apply this knowledge until after an accident has happened, the routine must be at your fingertips beforehand. There are several parts of the Help Routine which should be practised and memorized before an emergency occurs. (Giving the Kiss of Life, for example, only becomes difficult when you need to hold a book of instructions in your hand at the same time.) These routines are explained very simply in the Help Routine chapter, and occur again in the treatment sections.

Priorities

An important part of first aid is to recognize what is wrong; which condition, or which of several casualties, is to be given priority; what must be dealt with first and what may be left until later.

These are the basic priorities and in this order.

AIRWAY (breathing)

If the patient is not breathing he must be given artificial respiration immediately—usually the Kiss of Life.

BLEEDING

Serious bleeding must always have urgent treatment and is

second only to the restoration of breathing. Every effort must be made to stop the loss of blood.

CONSCIOUSNESS

An unconscious person is always in grave danger of having a blocked airway. The reason for unconsciousness must be sought and prompt action taken.

Remember these as your ABC priorities—airway, bleeding and consciousness—and always deal with these first. A broken bone, for example, provided it is not moved, will not suffer further if left for a short time while more pressing conditions receive attention.

So far we have mentioned four subjects dealt with in Section 1 of *Help!*: common causes of accidents, prevention of accidents, equipment for first aid and dealing with an emergency. The first two will help you to avoid emergencies; the last two will prepare you for emergencies when they happen.

The whole of Section 1 represents a mere one and a half to two hours' reading. When (not if, but when) you are faced with an emergency, you will be thankful you gave up this short time to be prepared.

One more condition that deserves priority mention is burns. They must be treated promptly, as swift action can minimize pain (which is often very severe) and prevent further damage.

Shock

It has not been necessary in *Help!* to treat shock as a separate subject, because it is associated with all injuries, but a word of explanation may be helpful. There are two kinds of shock—emotional shock and surgical shock.

Emotional shock occurs on the receipt of bad news or sometimes even good news. An unexpected telegram to say you have won the pools can be as disturbing to the emotions as the unexpected loss of a close relative. All that the 'patient' needs here is to be kept warm, be treated kindly, and perhaps be offered a cup of tea—never alcohol.

Surgical shock accompanies all illness or injury to a greater or lesser degree: the worse the condition, the worse the surgical shock will be. For example, the loss of blood will cause surgical shock. Stop the bleeding and you will stop the shock from getting worse. In hospital the blood can be replaced by transfusion and the shock should improve. So you will see that by treating the condition you are at the same time beginning to treat the shock.

Coping with confidence

One of the aims of *Help!* is simplicity, and first aid is a simple subject. As the name implies, first aid is aid given at the very first instant, correctly, quickly and gently, to save life and make the patient comfortable until he can be handed over to professional care—doctor, nurse, first aider or to an ambulance crew. The whole idea is to make sure that when handed over, the patient is no worse (if possible, better) than when you found him. This may even involve doing nothing at all for him, or certainly nothing that will aggravate his condition. Often you will find that good sound common sense will be your greatest ally. As a system, first aid has been greatly simplified in recent years, and you will find that all the courage you need to tackle emergencies will be given to you in the pages of this book.

You will notice two special symbols that appear in the margins throughout the text. A cross is used to indicate *treatments*, and the streaked cross is used where *medical aid* should be summoned urgently. In addition, each chapter has been identified with a chapter symbol which appears at the top outer corner of each page. Familiarise yourself with all these symbols and they will take you to the right page in an emergency without searching the index.

Help! gives instructions in plain language—no Latin names or technical terms—for dealing with all the common forms of accident likely to be sustained in the home and garden, on the road, and on holiday. Some treatments are general and apply to any part of the body. Other treatments are special, eg that for an injured eye.

And finally a few words of advice. Make sure all the family know where the first aid box is kept (out of reach of young children, but never under lock and key), and also where you keep this book (we suggest the book is kept with your first aid box). See that all the family read Section I of *Help!* as soon as possible. And keep calm at all times: with the aid of this book you will be capable and confident when an emergency arises.

Section 1

Being prepared

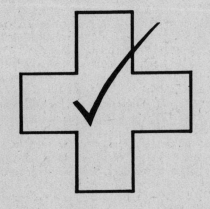

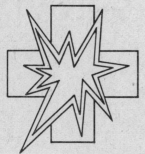

Chapter I

Accidents
~how they happen and how to avoid them

It would disappoint many readers if we didn't start this book with the time-honoured cliché, 'accidents don't just happen, they are caused.' So there it is, as large as life and just as true as it always was. Accidents continue to be caused by thoughtlessness, carelessness, neglect, and momentary lack of concentration; and alas it is not always the person who causes an accident who suffers: very often it is the innocent.

Why, it may be asked, do people lack concentration, thought and care? There may be many reasons. Tiredness, illness, stress, worry, anger, bad news and even good news or a celebration drink can all impair concentration and make you, temporarily, accident-prone. It is then that accidents are most likely to happen although, of course, they can happen at any time. There are also two age groups, the very old and the very young, who, by physical disability or lack of judgement, are a constant accident risk.

Just as an accident can happen at any time, it can also happen almost anywhere, provided hazards exist and there is activity. It is simple enough to identify such places in the home. The kitchen is the scene of most home accidents, because there is most activity here. Boiling liquids in kettles and saucepans, hot rings and oven bars, steam, electrical appliances, sharp knives (and even more dangerous, blunt ones—Fig. 1), are but a few of the kitchen hazards. Many home accidents also occur in the bathroom and on the staircase; and outside, in garden sheds or in the garage. (Why does the garage always collect so many poisons and inflammable materials?)

At work there is another whole range of danger points: in the factory there is a mass of mechanical and electrical equipment and possibly also dangerous substances such as chemicals; in the office there is electrical and other equipment, and there may be unsafe cupboards, filing cabinets, lifts and open staircases.

Then there are sports, all of which have certain elements of danger. Think of cricket and golf balls, football boots and hockey sticks, which can all leave their mark—or worse! Water sports, such as sailing, swimming and surfing, all have risks which can develop from simple situations into crises in a matter of seconds. Think again of the risks in rock climbing, pot-holing or hang-gliding, in which one slip can cost a life.

Fig. 1

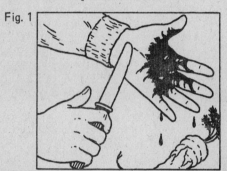

Travel also has its attendant dangers. In the field of public transport, higher speeds of planes and trains, introduced to save time, can result in greater and more serious emergencies. And for the motorist, the motorway network offers speed and ease as incentives, but takes its toll in multiple accidents when just one vehicle runs out of control, or sudden patches of mist or fog develop. Motoring danger is not restricted to motorways, however. Schools, shopping precincts and industrial centres are all places where a moment's preoccupation may mean tragedy.

Accidents caused by neglect are perhaps the most sinister of all. A faulty length of flex, or an imperfect appliance such as an electric blanket, may deteriorate very slowly to reach the critical moment at which a short circuit and fire occurs. No-one may be anywhere near the equipment at that second, and the fire may take hold strongly before it is noticed. There are dozens of places where such accidents are 'ripening'—waiting for the moment of action. A rung on a ladder, the brakes of a car, a hole in a carpet, a loose leg of a chair—these are but a few of the things that could be put right now to avoid certain disaster later.

If through extra care we eliminate the accident, we eliminate the suffering, hardship, inconvenience and the cost that it would have involved. Worthwhile? Definitely, you may say, especially if you have recently sustained an accident in the home, and can *measure* the suffering and cost. But what about next week's accident? Well, it may not be as soon as that, but it could be even sooner, and the cause may already be at work. Our duty to ourselves and our families is, firstly, to be efficient and so to prevent accidents from happening, and secondly, to know what to do when an accident does happen.

13

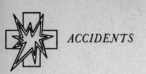

How to prevent accidents

Accident prevention is always better than first aid, and it has already been stressed that accidents are caused by carelessness, thoughtlessness and neglect. In this chapter, however, when we speak of cause, we shall be referring to the things that go wrong, not the people who allow them to happen. The causes of accidents are manifold and here it has been necessary to concentrate on those that happen most frequently. Practically all accidents fall into one of two groups: common accidents (which can happen almost anywhere) and particular accidents (which happen in a specific place or when using certain equipment).

Common accidents

Among the main causes of common accidents are electricity, gas, water, fire, and power-driven machinery.

ELECTRICITY

This can be a killer unless it is safely contained, and as a general rule people are far too careless with electricity. Here are some simple precautions.

1 Don't have unnecessarily long trailing leads on lamps and appliances. It is far safer to have plenty of wall sockets. Trailing leads soon become frayed, and frayed leads develop bare patches exposing wires which will cause electric shock, or short circuit leading in turn to fire. Trailing leads can be caught up by vacuum cleaners (Fig. 2), and they can trip people up.

Fig. 2

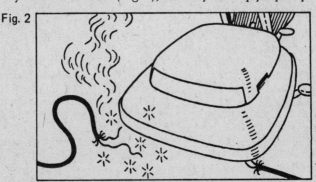

2 All appliances should have three-pin plugs. This ensures that the appliance is earthed via the wall socket, and not via your body. Always insert the appropriate fuse for the appliance in use (3, 5, 13 amp).

3 Don't overload lighting sockets by plugging high-wattage appliances into them or using adapters to carry excessive loads.

4 Never touch electric switches or appliances with wet hands: water is an excellent conductor of electricity.

5 Always switch off and disconnect plugs from sockets when appliances such as television, hi-fi equipment, electric fans, fires and mixers are not in use.

6 Electricity should not be turned off at the main switch when a house is to be empty for a period (eg during a holiday) if you are leaving a fridge or freezer containing food. A special inspection should therefore be made to ensure that everything else *is* switched off (especially cookers, electric blankets and the oil heater main switch).

7 Don't be a do-it-yourself bodger. Unless you are really competent at wiring plugs, making joints in lengths of flex and mending switches, leave it to the experts: in the end it is cheaper, and far safer.

GAS

Today there is considerable use of coal gas, natural gas and cylinder gases such as Calor gas. Some of them are poisonous and can cause death if inhaled in quantity, and all are highly explosive when mixed with air. The danger of gas-air mixtures is intensified by the fact that some are odourless, and all are colourless. There are a few precautions that will avoid the obvious dangers arising.

1 Check that all gas taps are properly turned off when not in use.

2 Never turn on a gas tap until you have matches or lighter in your hand.

3 If you smell gas, immediately turn off any gas flames or electric filament heaters (ie fires or cooking rings), and put out any naked lights and cigarettes. Do not seek the cause with a naked light.

4 Turn off at main before leaving house empty for a period (unless gas is serving refrigeration equipment), but make sure that all pilot lights are re-lit immediately after turning on again.

WATER

Inside the house or factory, water, just like electricity or gas, needs to be contained carefully in order to be safe; this applies to boiler equipment and calorifiers as well as cold water. Leaking water may not be noticed, but can soak through electrical equipment to cause short-circuit and fire, and this can happen at any time—perhaps at 3 o'clock in the morning when everyone is asleep.

Outside the home, water is found in garden ponds, lakes, streams and rivers, and of course, at the coast. The danger of drowning, especially among children and non-swimmers, is always present. Adults must be expected to take care of themselves, and to ask for information necessary for safe swimming and sailing. Children, however, and toddlers in particular, need protection from water, especially from garden ponds and swimming pools, which should be enclosed with fencing or wire netting during the toddling years.

FIRES

Open fires cause numerous emergencies every year. Damp wood which spits out sparks, or fires banked too high should always be guarded before retiring or when the room is empty. An efficient guard will also protect the very young and the old from falling into the fire.

Smoking, as a habit, can be regarded as a fire risk. Smokers occasionally manage (somehow!) to have two or even three cigarettes burning at the same time, and this can easily lead to fire. Always use ashtrays, and if a burning cigarette is balanced on the edge of an ashtray, it is safer to have the burning end outside the ashtray: then as it burns shorter, the butt will fall into the ashtray.

Some modern household materials are extremely inflammable, particularly polystyrene (used for ceiling tiles, modern furniture and packaging), and adhesives.

Bonfires are fun while roaring away, but they can be revived later on by a rising wind when no-one is there to watch them, and burning waste can be carried on the wind to start a fire. Bonfires and campfires should be beaten out, and inspected after an interval to ensure that they really *are* out.

POWER-DRIVEN MACHINERY

In the home this is restricted to equipment such as mixers, washing machines, spin driers, vacuum cleaners, fans and record or cassette players. In the office it may include duplicating, accounting and addressing equipment, as well as computer installations. In the factory, the worker is literally surrounded by electric motors, belt and other drives, and a mass of moving machinery. All are hazards. Government regulations put the onus on management and workers alike to see that working conditions are safe and healthy and that they are maintained. The employer is responsible for training employees (and himself) in the proper use of all equipment. Here are some tips for accident prevention:

1 Obey the rules—they were made for your protection.
2 Always wear the protective clothing appropriate to the job, such as goggles, helmets, overalls and gauntlets.
3 Never remove protective guards.
4 Never use a machine as a tool for any purpose other than its designed purpose.
5 Be careful with electricity—remember the dangers of an electric shock through wet hands and standing water, and of fire through overloading of sockets.
6 Always note carefully the position of main and controlling

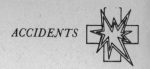

switches; a life often depends on the speed with which machinery is stopped.

Accidents room-by-room

KITCHEN

This is the place where most accidents happen, simply because it is the centre of activity and is full of hazards.

Knives

These are made sharp to cut food, not the cook. Always cut downwards onto a cutting board; never cut towards your hand. When carving meat, use a suitable sharp knife—it is less likely to slip than a blunt one—and hold the meat steady with a guarded fork.

Kitchen and utility room gadgets

Most modern households have washing machines, driers, mixers, shredders, liquidizers and other gadgets, and all have moving parts. Never put your fingers near these parts. Make sure that the socket is switched off before you plug in any of these gadgets, and dry your hands first.

Stoves and cookers

When in use all get extremely hot—that is what they are for. So don't touch the hot parts, and wear oven gloves when handling pots, pans, dishes and casseroles. Proper oven gloves are much safer than cloths, which can trail onto gas or electric rings, or into hot fat. A cloth may well prove too thin to protect against the heat and this may result in spilling, causing further burning. Handles of pots and saucepans are another hazard. Never leave them poking out into the kitchen, where they can be knocked: they should be positioned so that they protrude sideways, and are not over the cooker, where they may get hot and burn the hand (Fig. 3). When toddlers are around, it is safer always to use the back rings, which cannot be reached.

Fig. 3
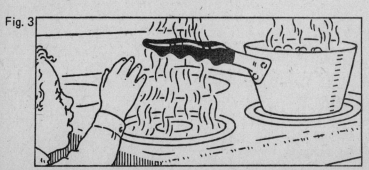

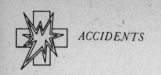
If a pan of fat catches fire, don't grab it and run for the garden; keep calm, turn off the ring under the pan (and any other rings that are on), and cover the pan with a *damp* cloth. This will immediately extinguish the flame. *On no account* pour water on a fat fire; the fat will 'explode' in your face, causing burns. Never keep aerosols near the cooker. Never pour hot liquids (eg fill a hot-water bottle) with your pet dog or cat at your feet.

Other hazards

Beware of teacloths that have extensive holes in them; they can cause breakages and if glass falls on the kitchen floor nasty cuts can result. When opening cans, always hold the can with a cloth. Cans have a habit of slipping and the jagged edge of a half-opened can may cause a deep cut. Polythene bags have a fascination for young children. Placed over the head they will quickly cause suffocation. Always keep them out of the way.

SITTING ROOM AND DINING ROOM

Even here accidents can happen: tea trays in the sitting room can be sent flying when dangling tablecloths are caught in shoes or are pulled by young children; such tablecloths should be avoided. In the dining room carving knives can slip causing cuts, and hot foods can be spilled while being served, causing burns or scalds. There is no simple rule for avoiding accidents of these kinds, except to take care, and work and move with a steady rhythm. When carving it is best not to push, but simply to do the sawing, and let the knife do the cutting. In this way it cannot slip.

STAIRCASE AND LANDING

These areas should be well lit, and should not be covered with worn-out or loose carpeting. Loose carpet on the staircase itself is extremely dangerous. Toys, shoes and other items which are 'on their way upstairs' often get dumped on the lower stairs. This is extremely dangerous, as anyone coming downstairs (especially if carrying a tray or basket) will trip over them and fall. Badly-fitting shoes and loose bedroom slippers are constantly causing accidents on the stairs. The hatchway into the roof area is usually positioned in the landing ceiling, and often access is by loose ladder or steps, or even by a tall stool placed under the hatchway. Never attempt to get up into the roof when you are alone in the house. If you fall and break a leg, you may be there all day without being able to attract attention.

BATHROOM AND WC

Make sure that the bathwater is not too hot, especially for children. Children always seem attracted to bathroom bottles and equipment. Razors, bleach and lavatory cleaners should be kept out of reach, and if the bathroom cabinet contains pills or

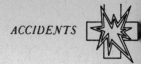

medicines it should be locked. Aerosol deodorants, shaving creams and hairsprays should be kept away from heat, and should *never* be thrown on a fire when empty. Hypothermia (excessive loss of body heat), strangely, is a danger for a very tired person taking a hot bath. Recently a woman in the prime of life died of hypothermia, simply through falling asleep in a hot bath and failing to wake before the water went cold. So if very tired, don't risk a hot bath if you are alone in the house, or if you bath, set an alarm clock! Never take sleeping pills with alcohol before taking a hot bath, for this will almost certainly induce sleep. Electricity is doubly dangerous in the bathroom. Switches should be of the corded type, and sockets (if any) must not be touched with wet hands. Government regulations forbid the fitting of standard sockets in bathrooms.

BEDROOMS

A few accidents are quite frequent in bedrooms. Electric fires used in winter will rapidly set the folds of diaphanous nightdresses and negligees on fire. It is a good rule never to dress children in nightdresses, but always in sleeping suits that fit neatly and snugly to the body.

Electric blankets need servicing from time to time, and it is extremely dangerous to have hot-water bottles and electric blankets in contact, for even a small leak from the hot-water bottle cap can cause a short-circuit and a fire. A bedside light — or light switch — will help to avoid the heavy bruising that can result from walking around in the dark and falling over or bumping into hard objects. It is extremely difficult to walk straight in a desired direction in the dark.

GARAGE AND GARDEN SHED

Garages are meant for cars, although a vast range of goods and chattels usually manages to accumulate there. Always drive the car into and out of your garage with extra care. Especially when reversing you should make sure no-one is behind you: remember that your vision is very restricted. If petrol and paraffin must be kept in the garage, keep them away from the track used by the car and from the area used when the car doors are opened. Never store inflammable or poisonous materials in squash or mineral bottles which children will tend to drink from, and keep them where they are safe from fire.

Mowers and garden tools, axes, and rusty nails in old pieces of wood can all cause jagged wounds; and, in inexperienced hands, saws, chisels, drills and power tools are all potential hazards. Weed-killers and insecticides can be poisonous if swallowed, and some can be skin irritants, so they should be kept where they are safe, and away from children. Strong acids and alkalis can give bad burns and should be similarly isolated.

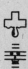

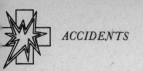

Modern adhesives

Many shops and stores are now selling a new 'super-glue' (cyanoacrylate adhesive) which is very fast setting and extremely strong. If it comes in contact with the skin it will firmly bond two skin surfaces together. Provided the following method is carried out carefully, there should be no injury, but *do not* try to pull the skin surfaces apart, for you will only tear away the skin.

ADHESIVE ON THE FINGERS

A Immerse the stuck surfaces in warm soapy water.
B Gently and carefully peel or roll the surfaces apart, using a teaspoon handle or a spatula.
C Remove the adhesive from the skin with soap and water.

ADHESIVE IN THE EYE

A Wash the eyelid or eyeball thoroughly with warm water.
B Cover the eye with a dressing.
The eye will open in one to four days without further action, but if you are at all concerned, seek medical advice. Excessive tear formation or double vision may be experienced for several hours, but there is no chronic after-effect.

ADHESIVE IN THE MOUTH

It is almost impossible to swallow the adhesive, as it forms a lump in the mouth.
A If the lips are stuck use plenty of warm water or use your spit.
B Gently peel or roll the lips apart.
When a large quantity of adhesive comes in contact with the skin, heat may be released as it hardens, causing burns. In such cases, first remove the adhesive with warm soapy water, and then treat as for burns.

Sports and hobbies

There is an element of danger in many games. Balls, bats and rackets, boots, and even opponents, can prove to be very hard indeed. Sports injuries can be minimized by obeying the rules, taking no risks, and checking and maintaining the condition of the equipment used. These rules are paramount in the more challenging sports such as pot-holing, water ski-ing, white water canoeing, parachuting and hang-gliding. The rules are still applicable, and indeed necessary, in the case of conventional games, such as football, cricket and tennis.

Generally there will be a first aid box and equipment wherever organized sport is held, but it is always well to ask if it does in fact exist. If you are instrumental in having it provided, you will have done a good turn for others, and perhaps yourself.

Fig. 4

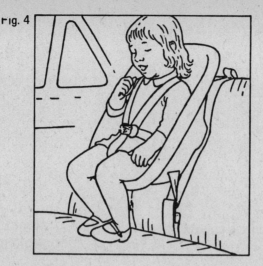

On the road

Using the public highway, whether in public transport, in a car or on a bicycle, has attendant hazards. Many of them can be avoided by your own good care. The best advice that can be given here is to know and obey the rules of the road.

Always use seat belts. Children in cars should always be belted to the back seat, or to a special child's seat (Fig. 4), fixed to the back seat. Be careful when shutting car doors; fingers caught in them can be most painful. Frequently one or more fingernails may be lost as a result, and it takes several months of constant annoyance before this finally happens. Never 'hold' a car on a hill by using the clutch, for this may dislocate a hip or cause pains in the back; use the handbrake, and relax. Finally, see that your car has adequate petrol and oil, radiator and battery water, and check tyre pressures including the spare. The moment of failure which may result from neglect of these simple check-ups is sure to be highly inconvenient, and may possibly be dangerous to boot. On long journeys where you may be some distance from service stations always carry adequate emergency supplies of water, petrol and oil.

Pedestrians should wear light clothing at night, carry a torch, and walk on the side of the road facing approaching traffic. Children and cyclists should wear reflective or fluorescent clothing or bands.

Summary

The suggestions we have made here for avoiding accidents are no more than examples of sensible prudent behaviour for good living, free from worry. Each rule or tip is the result of thought, care and concentration taken by others before us. If you can follow them and avoid taking unnecessary risks, your life will be safer. Don't think 'it can't happen to me'—because it can, and it might.

Chapter 2

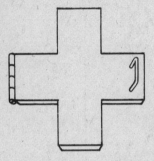

Equipment

A certain amount of first aid equipment is a necessity, although here we have been careful to keep cost to a minimum. It is essential that a first aid box is kept in the home and a smaller one in the car. Together their contents are not expensive, and the cost is truly justifiable.

For the home

A first aid box can be made out of a clean biscuit tin or a large plastic container. The box should be clearly labelled 'first aid', with a red cross, and should be lined with absorbent kitchen paper. The lid, when removed and covered with a piece of absorbent kitchen paper, provides a clean working surface. Whatever you choose as a first aid box, it must be easily carried and on no account should it be screwed to the wall. The best site is in the kitchen. Unfortunately most accidents in the home occur here anyway, and it is also quite a good place to carry out first aid treatment. Wherever it is kept, all the family must know where to find it, and on no account should it be locked up. It must be kept out of reach of young children, however.

Once equipment has been used, the box must be topped up and replaced in its correct place. Don't say to yourself 'I'll do it later'—tomorrow never comes. It will not get done, and you will be caught out in an emergency. Also remember not to get your usual household lotions and potions mixed up with your first aid box, which must contain purpose equipment only. The various medicines and tablets prescribed by your family doctor should not be hoarded anyway. Surplus pills and liquids should be returned to the chemist or flushed down the lavatory. Grandpa's cough medicine is valueless to anyone else and may actually be harmful. Even medicines kept specifically for emergencies should be stored separately from the first aid box, possibly in a bathroom cupboard away from children. So here are three lists—

One for the home first aid box.
One for the bathroom cupboard.
One for the car.

FIRST AID BOX IN THE HOME

1 Three (or more) triangular bandages (commonly called slings). These can be used to keep dressings in place, as a sling to support an injured arm, to apply pressure when a casualty is bleeding and to restrict movement when a fracture is suspected.

2 Three each small, medium and large sterile emergency dressings. These are packaged sterile dressings made of wool and gauze or lint, with bandages attached, that are used to cover the more serious wounds in an emergency until further medical care is available.

3 Selection of adhesive dressings for minor cuts, wounds or grazes.

4 Supply of cotton wool balls. These have many uses, such as swabbing, drying or cleaning wounds. They are best kept in a polythene bag.

5 A suitable antiseptic, for cleaning dirty minor wounds. Cetavlon BP is useful, but soap and water is more than adequate. Always read instructions on the bottle of antiseptic most carefully, and use a small container (an egg cup or a clean tin-foil pie dish) for diluting and preparing the antiseptic for use.

6 Small packet of sterile gauze squares.

7 Adhesive plaster.

8 Cotton conforming bandages 2″ and 3″ (approximately 5 cm and 7½ cm).
Items 6, 7 and 8 are used to cover and retain dressings to minor wounds that do not require medical treatment.

9 Clean square of white linen—an old sheet is ideal, when cleaned, ironed well, aired and placed in a polythene bag. This is torn to size and used to cover burns and scalds after treatment, or may be placed under an injured limb to protect clothing.

10 Paper and pencil to record clues including pulse rate.

11 Useful additions include a packet of tissues, a supply of small polythene bags (for soiled dressings and vomit), kitchen paper for mopping up blood and vomit or providing a clean working surface, safety pins and scissors (with blunt ends).

THE MEDICINE CUPBOARD (out of reach of children)

1 A suitable preparation for relief of minor pain, headaches and toothache. If pain or headache persists, go to your doctor for

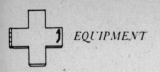

advice. Pain is often nature's way of saying something else is wrong, Paracetamol B.P. or its equivalent may be used.

2 A preparation for indigestion and stomach upsets. Most families have their favourites, but a chemist will advise. A glass of milk will often be sufficient.

3 Calamine lotion or cream for the relief of sunburn, bites and rashes, or other skin irritations.

4 Hot lemon drinks, now available, are excellent for resisting coughs and colds in their developing stages.

5 Tablets for travel sickness—especially if there are known sufferers in the home. But do read the directions carefully.

First aid box in the car

Always carry a small box, marked with a red cross in a white circle, containing

1 Six triangular bandages.

2 Three each small, medium and large emergency dressings.

3 Safety pins and scissors (with blunt ends).

4 Small packet assorted adhesive dressings.

5 Small polythene bags for vomit, false teeth if removed, and personal belongings.

6 Packet of tissues for mopping and cleaning.

7 Paper and pencil for recording clues and casualty's name and address.

8 Useful extras include rug or blanket, and torch.

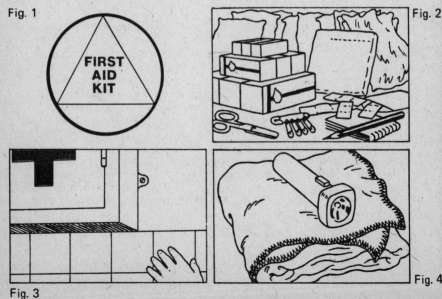

Fig. 1

FIRST AID KIT

Fig. 2

Fig. 3

Fig. 4

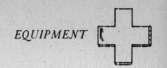

When this equipment is carried in your car, it is useful to display a disc stating that a first aid kit is carried. Such discs (Fig. 1) are available at stores selling motor equipment or from the stores department of your Ambulance Association. All the equipment listed here may be bought at any chemist's, or again through the stores department of your Ambulance Association. The recommended equipment is illustrated in Figs. 2, 3 and 4.

Applying the triangular bandage

These bandages can be made of linen, or there is a cheaper disposable (but inflammable) type. They can be made out of old sheets, provided they are cut from a 90 cm (36″) square, cut diagonally. Figure 5 shows how the bandage is applied.

AS AN ARM SLING

To rest or support an injured arm:
A Place point under injured elbow (Fig. 6).

Fig. 5

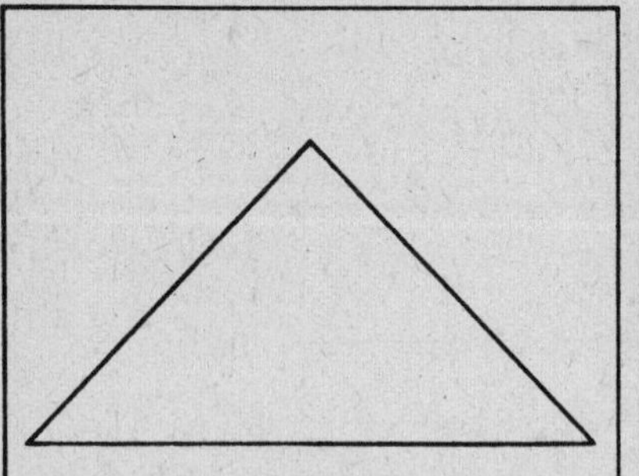

Fig. 6

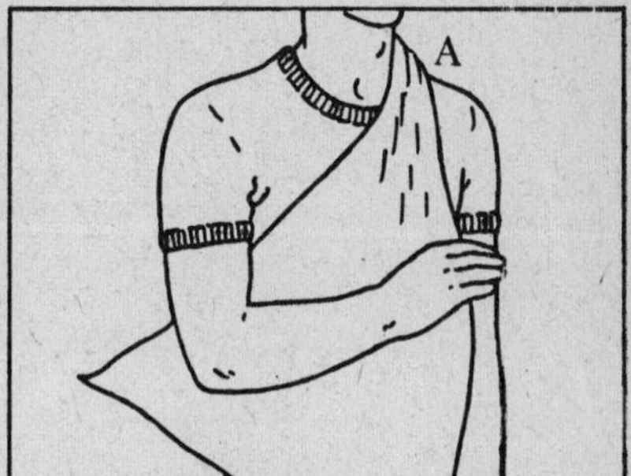

Fig. 7

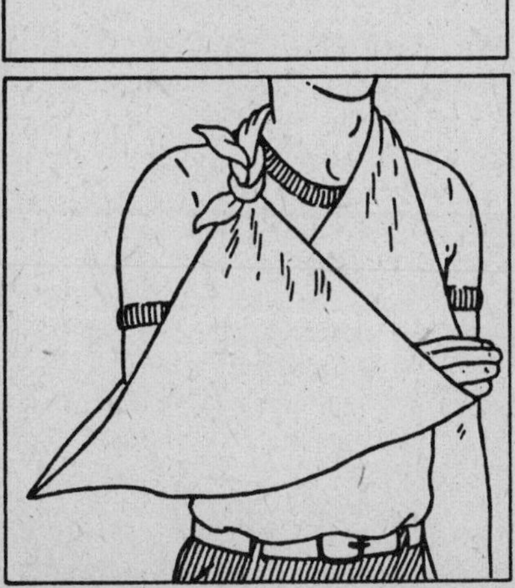

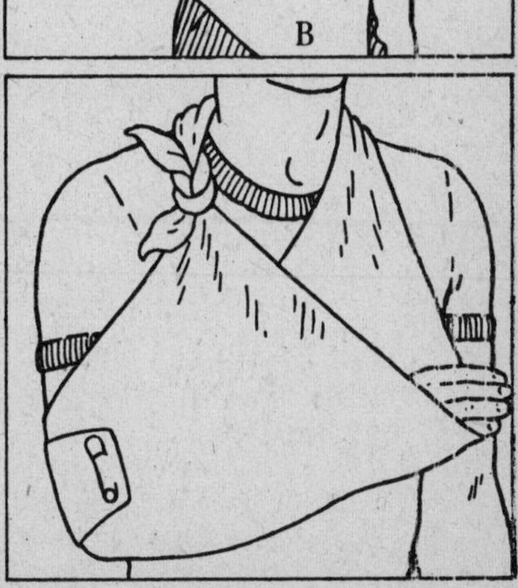

Fig. 8

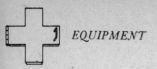

Fig. 9

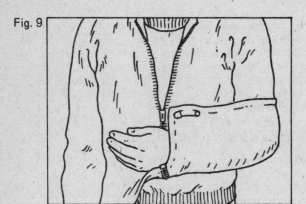

Fig. 10

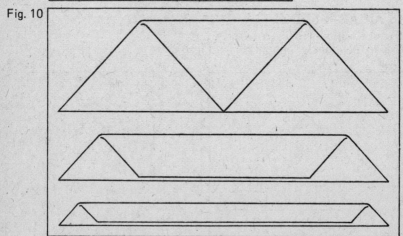

B Take end A around back of neck.
C Bring end B up to A and tie together on the injured shoulder, using a reef knot (Fig. 7), which will not slip and is better than a 'granny'.
D Bring point (at elbow) to front and secure with a safety pin, forming a pocket to support the elbow (Fig. 8).

When completed the arm should be comfortable, resting just above the average belt-line. The wrist should not dangle. There may be times when no triangular bandage is available and then you must improvise. Here are one or two ideas:
A Use a headscarf or a belt to make a sling.
B The hand or forearm can be tucked inside a buttoned-up coat or firm cardigan.
C The bottom of an anorak or cardigan can be turned up and the

hem secured to the main body of the garment with a safety-pin, forming a sling (Fig. 9).
If you improvise, you must be quite certain that the limb is comfortable and held securely.

OTHER USES OF THE TRIANGULAR BANDAGE

As we have said, the triangular bandage has many uses and you will find it is mentioned several times as you read on. It may be folded into a narrow bandage (Fig. 10), and like this it may be used:
A To support limbs (Fig. 11).
B To hold a dressing in place (Fig. 12).
C Applied firmly, to control bleeding (as Fig. 12).
D Folded as a broad bandage, to give extra support (as Fig. 11).

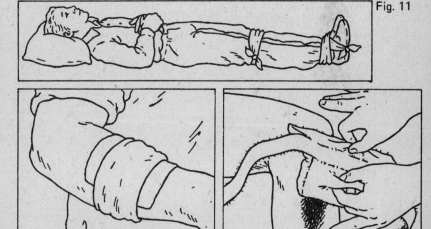

Fig. 11

Fig. 12

Fig. 13

Applying compressed dressings

A Using the tab provided, carefully remove the outer wrapping. This will probably reveal a further protective coat of paper to keep the dressing sterile.
B Tear open this wrapper, and carefully remove the tightly folded dressing, holding it by the bandaged area. Unwind the bandage and two ends appear.
C At all times handle only the bandage. Your fingers should *never* touch the inside of the dressing, which is sterile (Fig. 13). Now place the inside of the dressing on the wound and bandage firmly but not too tightly, winding the ends of the bandage around the dressing, and making sure that the dressing is held firmly and comfortably in position.

27

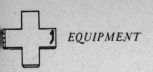

Once again, there will be occasions when a compressed dressing is not available, and here are a few substitutes.
1 Paper or linen handkerchiefs.
2 Old linen.
3 Paper kitchen towels.
4 Any clean and smooth material—fabrics that have been recently ironed are particularly useful.
Just remember that whatever you use should be large enough to cover the wound and it is most important to handle the makeshift dressing as little as possible and *never* touch the side that will be applied to the wound.

Applying conforming bandages

If you buy the cotton conforming bandages recommended in the first aid kit, which stretch and mould themselves to the irregular and tapering shapes of the body, you will not need to learn complicated bandaging techniques (Fig. 14).

Fig. 14
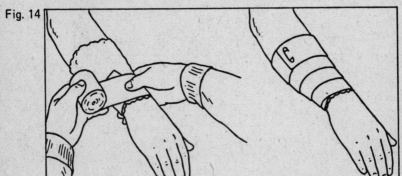

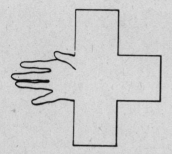

Chapter 3

Taking action

The first thing you must do before you can help anyone else is to organize yourself. To handle an accident, therefore, it is essential to make the most of your limited skill, equipment, and time. This is easiest when reduced to a routine. In this way you are more likely to keep a clear head and do what is necessary in a precise and logical order. This is what we call the Help Routine. (The complete Help Routine provides for accidents *anywhere*, and therefore for accidents in the home you will need to modify the instructions. For instance you will know where your telephone is without looking for it.)

The preliminary routine

A Never panic or get in a flap.

B Go quickly but calmly to the scene of the accident. Don't run and arrive shaking and breathless.

C Remember to take the first aid box with you—this will save time and you can avoid leaving the casualty unattended.

D When you arrive try to size up the situation at a glance look carefully but quickly and note as much detail as you can. This can help you to understand what might have happened—but don't jump to hasty conclusions until you have made a fuller examination.

A special treatment of road accidents is given in Chapter 12. If more than one casualty needs help, decide on the order of treatment, from most to least serious. Look around for help, and remember helpful people may need telling what to do. Look also for a telephone and note any useful equipment for improvisation.

E Guard against further danger to the casualty and yourself.

F If there is anyone to ask, find out what has happened (doctors call this the history).

G Look especially for a medic alert bracelet on the casualty's

Fig. 1

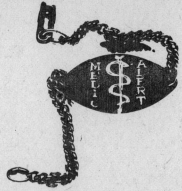

wrist (Fig. 1). If there is one, this should be advised to the
hospital when calling for emergency services.

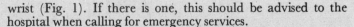

H Emergency services should now be contacted, if there is a helper
available to do so. But remember it is more important to save
the life of a casualty who has stopped breathing than to call for
help.

The emergency services routine

Handing a casualty over to professional aid is called disposal.
Whilst it would seem logical that you would first examine your
casualty, next diagnose his condition and finally carry out the
treatment before thinking of disposal, you should nevertheless
think ahead in the case of serious injuries where extra help is
going to be needed, and call for or send for it as early as possible.
If therefore you feel that the casualty's injury or condition is such
that hospital is essential, or that a doctor would send the casualty
on to hospital, telephone for help immediately, or get someone to
do so for you. With a little forethought it is possible to give the
authorities the precise information they need in a few words. The
procedure is:

A *Before* telephoning, have an address which will identify the
scene of the accident, ready to give to the authorities.

B Dial 999 or ask operator for 'Emergency services'.

C If ambulance, police and fire (rescue) services are required, ask
for them all at the same time.

D Give an indication of the number of casualties.

E Give any helpful information on nature and seriousness of
injuries sustained; this information can be life-saving.

In the case of minor injuries the casualty, having received your
treatment, probably needs no more than reassuring words and a
cup of tea, with arrangements being made for him to get home—
if he is not there already. It might also be wise to see that his
family doctor is advised of the accident and the treatment. But if
in your opinion skilled medical help is still necessary after first aid,
it is best to get the casualty to his family doctor if possible, though

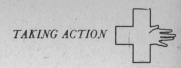

if too far from home, hospital is the alternative, and you should use the emergency services routine just described.

The examination

With the situation now under control and emergency services (where appropriate) duly alerted, the next stage is the examination of the injured. Always start where it hurts, or in the case of an unconscious casualty, at the head. Where unconsciousness is suspected, test for it as follows:

THE SHAKE, SHOUT AND PINCH ROUTINE

Try to rouse the casualty by these three methods, and in this order. If the casualty does not respond to shaking, shouting and pinching he can be diagnosed as unconscious, and must immediately be treated according to the priority routines referred to later in this chapter under 'treatment' (see page 33).

THE SEE, HEAR AND FEEL ROUTINE

This is a comprehensive but simple system for spotting clues which can be put together to help make a final diagnosis of the casualty's injuries. In the coloured casualty it is sometimes difficult to notice changes, especially in the colour of the skin. Guidance on these changes is given on page 38. Proceed in this order:

A If the casualty can talk, ask what is wrong and where it hurts (doctors call these the symptoms). Start your examination where it hurts.

B If the casualty cannot talk—he may be unconscious or paralysed—start looking for clues (doctors call these the signs) in the following order. Learn to recognize these clues easily—they will be explained later.

C Always start with the head, for here you may find a lot of important clues, such as:
Breathing: or not breathing, fast or slow, quietly or noisily, unusual smells on breath.
Scalp: examine the scalp for wounds, bleeding, bumps or swellings. Look carefully, and feel gently (remember that hair may hide some of these symptoms).
Face: the colour may be red (flushed), white (pale) or blue (cyanosed), the skin may be hot or cold and it may be dry or damp.
Eyes: large or small pupils (or even one large and one small).
Mouth: fluids may be discharged, coughed or vomited.
Nose: look for discharge.
Ears: look for discharge.
Blood or pale-coloured fluid—or a mixture of both—may come from the mouth, nose or ear.

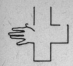

D *The pulse*

The pulse, or heart-beat, can be felt wherever an artery comes close to the body's surface, but it is more easily taken at the wrist (Fig. 2) or neck. It may be absent altogether, or its speed and strength may vary. Speed is described as slow, normal or fast, and strength as feeble, normal or full (pounding).

Fig. 2

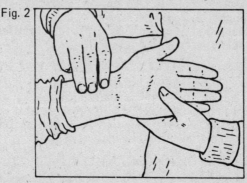

E *The body and limbs*

Bleeding: Look for bleeding but not only from obvious wounds. Feel clothing for any damp, sticky patches. Blood may also come from the natural holes—from the back passage or passed with urine.

Swellings, bumps and lumps: These unusual features may indicate that something is wrong under the surface of the body. (Remember that some people do have rather odd bumps, like knobbly knees, though most of us are approximately the same each side. And some natural curves, especially in women, can vary considerably: the *unnatural* ones are painful to touch!). Therefore you should compare one side of the body with the other and note irregularities carefully.

It is easy to find clues when they come out to meet you, but internal damage—serious damage to the organs in the chest or belly, or to muscles, bones and joints—must be sought.

The diagnosis

After making a full examination of the patient and recording a set of clues (the signs and symptoms in doctor's language), you should be led on to a conclusion of what is wrong. This is called the diagnosis and only when your diagnosis has been made can you start the treatment. Do not think from reading this chapter that by the time you get to the diagnosis your casualty will be beyond help. You will be amazed at your quick response to an emergency, and the basic treatment for specific injuries and conditions in the following chapters will tell you how to proceed.

The treatment

Only when an accident has actually happened will you need to
refer to Section II of *Help!*, for there the chapters deal with the
treatment for all the common forms of injury sustained in
accidents. There are however, three priorities (to which we have
already referred) and three life-saving routines which occur over
and over again in Section II, and it is always these on which you
should concentrate first in an emergency. Learn, understand and
practise them *now* and you will double your usefulness in an
emergency. (Not only you but all the family should do this.)
The priorities apply to treatment for failure to breathe, heavy loss
of blood, unconsciousness, burns and scalds, broken bones,
poisons, bites and stings, road accident injuries, holiday and
sports injuries, as well as the everyday wounds we are all familiar
with. Here they are.

THE PRIORITIES

Attending immediately to the three basic priorities—airway,
bleeding and consciousness—guarantees that the casualty's life is
not going to slip through your fingers. Of course he may be
beyond help (and this is no fault of yours) but he *may not*. So
always proceed to check these priorities first, and *in this order*:

A *Airway (breathing)*: If the patient is not breathing he must be
 made to breathe at once: however bad his general condition
 this comes first, for without breathing life ceases in a matter of
 minutes. The casualty must be given the Kiss of Life immediately.

B *Bleeding*: Serious loss of blood is extremely dangerous and has
 overall priority once the casualty is breathing properly. The
 dressing of wounds is covered in detail in Chapter 5. At all
 costs serious bleeding must be stopped.

C *Consciousness*: Loss of consciousness is fraught with danger
 and needs urgent attention. To ensure continued breathing
 the casualty's head must be turned into a position in which the
 passage to his lungs cannot be blocked by his tongue, his saliva,
 his vomit or his blood. If you leave an unconscious casualty on
 his back gazing up to heaven he will soon be there to see for
 himself! It takes just a moment to turn the casualty's head to
 one side and to tip the chin up and the forehead back. Once this
 has been done, the casualty's continued breathing must be
 checked periodically. Should you hear a noise or gurgling in
 the mouth or throat the casualty must instantly be turned into
 the Recovery Position. If you remember nothing else but can
 place an unconscious casualty in the Recovery Position you
 have a better chance of keeping him alive until professional
 help arrives. On a hot day erect some kind of shelter against
 the sun.

THE RECOVERY POSITION

A Turn the casualty onto his back.
B Tuck the left arm under the left buttock.
C Place the right arm above the head (Fig. 3)
D Pull the body over on top of the left side.
E Bend the right leg up to the bent position.
F Bend the right arm into the bent position (Fig. 4).
G Ease the left arm out behind the body.
H Clear away anything loose from the mouth and throat, including dentures, to produce a clear airway.
I Now lift the head upwards and backwards to ensure that the airway is clear (Fig. 5).

Fig. 3

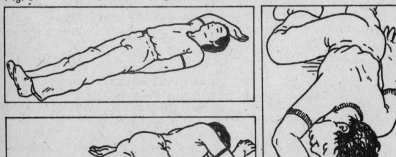

Fig. 5

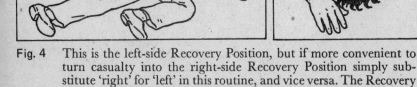

Fig. 4 This is the left-side Recovery Position, but if more convenient to turn casualty into the right-side Recovery Position simply substitute 'right' for 'left' in this routine, and vice versa. The Recovery Position routine is repeated in Chapter 6.

THE KISS OF LIFE ROUTINE or Mouth to Mouth breathing

A If it is possible to get someone else to call an ambulance, this is the first thing you arrange, but every second counts and you do *not* have time to do this yourself. If there is no-one to do this for you, it must wait until the patient has received first aid.
B Turn the casualty, when possible, so that he is lying on his back.
C Loosen clothing round casualty's neck, chest and waist, clean his mouth and nose, and remove any dentures, vomit, food or saliva, using a tissue or handkerchief over your fingers.
D Place one of your hands under the neck and the other on the forehead so that the casualty's head is tilted backwards (Fig. 6).

34

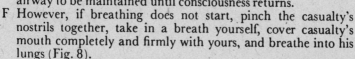

E Using the hand from under the neck, lift the chin upwards (Fig. 7). This simple procedure often clears the airway, when the casualty will take a breath and start to breathe on his own. But it is important to keep the head in this position for the clear airway to be maintained until consciousness returns.

F However, if breathing does not start, pinch the casualty's nostrils together, take in a breath yourself, cover casualty's mouth completely and firmly with yours, and breathe into his lungs (Fig. 8).

G From the corner of your eye you will see his chest rise; remove your mouth and turn your head away, and the chest will fall (casualty breathing out).

Fig. 6

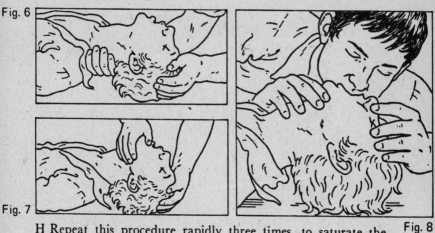

Fig. 7

Fig. 8

H Repeat this procedure rapidly three times, to saturate the casualty's blood with oxygen, then continue the procedure regularly, at the rate of about twelve times a minute. To pace yourself, here is a useful gimmick. *In your mind*, keep repeating the following jingle at a lively rate:

> *Turn head, breathe in, turn back,*
> *Breathe out: I've got the knack*.

I If the chest fails to rise, make sure that the head is tilted well back and the air passages are clear, and start again.

You should continue to give the Kiss of Life until the casualty breathes unaided. Then, if you have been unable to summon help or send for an ambulance earlier, you can arrange yourself for an ambulance to get the casualty to hospital.

For children and infants use the same routine, but remember the following points:

A Your mouth may be placed over both mouth and nose of the child.

B Breathe out more gently into the child.

The Kiss of Life routine is repeated in Chapter 4.

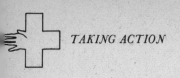
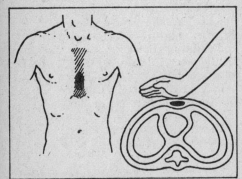

Fig. 9

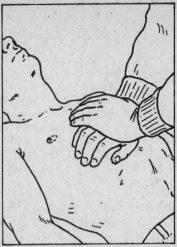

Fig. 10

HEART MASSAGE ROUTINE

If a casualty is unconscious he should be examined to make certain his heart is still beating. If it is not, you will see blueness in the lids of the eyes, dilated pupils, and there will be no pulsation in the neck or chest. Now you must immediately start heart massage, but remember heart massage must *never* be carried out on anyone whose heart has not in fact stopped, so always check first. Even when practising heart massage, a dummy should be used—*never* a person. This is the routine:

A The casualty must be lying on the ground or a hard surface.

B Turn the casualty onto his back, as if looking up to the sky.

C Kneel at one side of the chest (the most convenient side giving you the most room to move about).

D Find the lower half of the breastbone (the bone to which the ribs are joined in the front of the chest (Fig. 9).

E Place the heel of the right hand on the lower half of the breastbone.

F Place the left hand on top of the right (Fig. 10).

G With your arms straight push vertically down on the lower half of the breastbone for about 4 cm (1½″) in the adult.

H Repeat the pressure between 60–70 times a minute for adults; for children the rate is 80–90 per minute and you push the chest down about 2½ cm (1″); for infants the rate is 90–100 per minute and you gently push the chest down about 1 cm (½″). The rhythm of the pressure down should always be as regular and even as possible.

If your treatment is being given correctly you will quickly see an improvement in the colour of the casualty, ie the blueness will disappear and the pupils will return to normal size.

You will also start to see the pulsations in the neck again, and you will be able to hear the heart-beat in the chest. The See, Hear and Feel routine will tell you that your treatment is successful.

If you happen to be alone with a casualty when his heart and breathing stops, you are still able to carry out the Kiss of Life and

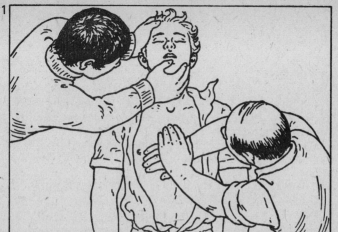

Fig. 11

heart massage as described, but you have to remember to alternate the giving of each. The rate is two quick chest inflations (two Kiss of Life) to fifteen presses (fifteen heart massage).

If you are fortunate to have a companion with you, first call an ambulance and then one of you can carry out the Kiss of Life and the other, heart massage (Fig. 11). The rate then is one Kiss of Life to five presses (heart massage). The heart massage routine is repeated in Chapter 4.

The coloured casualty

The diagnosis of shock or cyanosis (blueness) in a coloured casualty is not always as easy as in the white, but nevertheless there are certain signs that will appear.

SHOCK

There is of course no difference anatomically between coloured people and white, except for the colour of the skin. So all the signs of shock will appear in the coloured casualty in just the same way as in the non-coloured; but it is difficult to note pallor of the skin when the skin is dark brown or near black. The clues to look for are:

1 Cold clammy skin.
2 Rapid pulse (100 or more).
3 Rapid shallow breathing.
4 Feeling of nausea.
5 Dryness of lips and mouth.
6 Pallor of the skin will show in the palms of the hands and pads of the fingers.
7 The lips, and just inside the lips, will go pale.
8 The inside of the lower eyelids, when gently pulled down, will be pale.
9 The shine on the skin will disappear, making it look dull like a matt finish.
10 In severe shock, dilation of the pupils will occur.

37

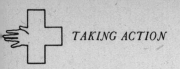

CYANOSIS

In a white casualty, cyanosis or blueness is easily seen by the blueness of the lips, lobes of the ears, finger nails and toe nails.

In the coloured casualty it is necessary to look for clues in the same places as for shock:

1 The lips, and just inside the lips, will appear blue.
2 The inside of the lower eyelids, when gently pulled down, will be blue.
3 The palms and the nail beds of the fingers and toes will be blue.
4 The coloured skin will lose its shine and go a matt blue-grey colour.

Conclusion

All that has been included in this chapter may seem a bewildering list of things to look for and do, and you may be thinking 'I'll never do it'. But sooner or later the situation may be thrust upon you without option, and you will *have* to do something. So don't run away! By learning the simple, calm approach of the Help Routine, you may one day save unnecessary pain and suffering, and even life.

Summary of the Help Routine

Reduced to the following simple instructions:

1 Don't panic.
2 Go to where help is needed.
3 Take your first aid box with you.
4 Size up situation.
5 Don't take any risks.
6 Prevent further injury to your casualty (and yourself).
7 Send for emergency services as considered necessary.
8 If casualty is conscious ask where it hurts.
9 If casualty is unconscious, check: Is he breathing?
   If breathing, maintain a clear airway.
   If not, give Kiss of Life immediately.
   If no pulse, give heart massage immediately.
10 Look for bleeding, and treat.
11 Make detailed examination of casualty.
12 Summarize clues.
13 Make your diagnosis.
14 Treat as appropriate—treat burns, cover wounds, immobilize fractures.
15 Check on arrangements for transit to hospital, doctor or home.

Continuing care

First aid entails more than initial treatment of the casualty. When handed over to professional care he must be no worse for your treatment, and preferably he should be better.

Never leave your casualty when help is on the way: you can still do valuable work. Observe any change in his condition. For example if blood soaks through the dressing you have just applied, another dressing will need to be applied, *on top of* the original dressing. There is also the possibility that the casualty is losing consciousness. You can tell by careful observation. The ambulance men will need whatever information you can give them, so *write down* anything that you believe to be relevant or important and hand it to them on their arrival.

Here is an example:

John Smith aged 11 years
Date 1st January 19...
12 noon John fell off bike and hit his head
12.10 John drowsy—can't give his name
12.20 Can't rouse him
12.25 Arrival of ambulance

(In this particular example, your ongoing care would have led you to turn John into the Recovery Position).

Pulse rate

It can often be quite useful to count and record a casualty's pulse rate. It is of little value to do this however if you don't write it down, so that the information is passed on. The pulse rate that becomes slower or faster is significant, and may indicate bleeding or other conditions.

The pulse can best be felt in the wrist (Fig. 2, page 32). The right place is found on the thumb side about 1 cm ($\frac{1}{2}$") from the line where the lower arm and palm of hand join. Place your first three fingers on this area, and roll your fingers until you feel the beat distinctly. Then count for a full minute. This may require a little practice.

The normal pulse rate is 60–80 beats per minute for adults, 90–100 for children, and 100–140 for infants. A record of pulse readings might appear thus:

Mary Jones, aged 7 years
Date 1st July 19...
11.00 fell off swing—large painful area over
left abdomen—very pale
11.15 pulse 94 beats
11.25 pulse 106 beats
11.35 pulse 120 beats
11.45 pulse 132 beats
11.50 arrival of ambulance

In this case Mary probably has internal haemorrhage, action is necessary, and the information collected is vital.

Shock

Next is the question of shock. You will recall that this accompanies all accidents in greater or lesser degree. If casualty becomes cold and shivery, this is a symptom. But do not react by piling blankets on the casualty or surrounding him with hot water bottles. One blanket over the patient is adequate, and one underneath him if you consider it is safe and possible to move him. Once again, children and the elderly need special care at times of crisis: they need more careful explanation and reassurance than fit adults do when similarly injured.

Shock can take some time to develop, so after an accident try to ensure that the casualty rests. The accident may not merit hospital treatment, but the casualty must still be made to lie down for a while—it need not be in bed. Children, in fact, settle better on a sofa in the sitting room where they can see what is going on— but remember rest somewhere is imperative while the body itself starts to repair the damage done.

Well-meaning onlookers will often rush forward to give the casualty brandy (or any other alcoholic drink they happen to have with them). But it is far more likely to do harm than good, and the safe rule is therefore *never* in any circumstances give alcohol.

Conscious casualties find nothing more discouraging than hearing bystanders discussing sport, politics and local gossip as though they were not there at all. Do please talk to casualties and help keep their minds off their plight. There is no need to talk about their injuries, but they will be able to relax a little if they realise that you have the situation in hand and that you will do for them what they cannot do for themselves, such as telephoning relatives. This applies particularly to road accidents.

Section II

Routines
for giving assistance

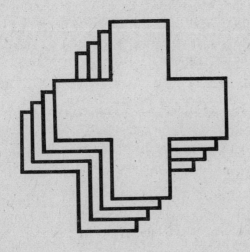

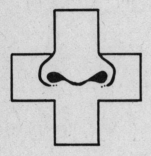

Chapter 4

Breathing

Breathing is the process by which air is drawn into the chest through the nose and mouth and is then blown out again through the same passages. Whilst in the chest, or more precisely the lungs, the air gives up some of its oxygen (about 1/5th) and this is taken into the blood circulation; in return the blood gives up the same amount of its waste product, carbon dioxide. This process is a continuous one from the time of birth to the time of death, and is often visible and obvious. If breathing stops, then within three or four minutes the heart will fail. Every second counts therefore, and in an emergency first read the summary on page 49 (The symptoms and treatment of heart failure are included in this chapter, but first things first.) How do you know if someone is not breathing? You carry out the See, Hear and Feel routine.

LOOK AND SEE
The chest wall will not be moving up and down.
The stomach wall will not be moving in and out.

LISTEN
You will not hear air being drawn in or blown out through the nose or mouth or into and out of the lungs, when you place your ear near the casualty.

FEEL
Your hand will not move up and down when placed on the chest. If you see nothing, hear nothing and feel nothing, then the casualty is not breathing.
    Once you have decided this you must start artificial breathing or artificial respiration immediately. The Kiss of Life (mouth-to-mouth resuscitation) is the simplest and recommended method, and artificial respiration is only used in special cases, to which we refer later. The aim of the Kiss of Life is to do the work of breathing when the casualty cannot do it himself.

The Kiss of Life routine

A If it is possible to get someone else to call an ambulance, this is the first thing you arrange, but every second counts and you do *not* have time to do this yourself. If there is no-one to do this for you, it must wait until the patient has received first aid.

B Turn the casualty, when possible, so that he is lying on his back.

C Loosen clothing round casualty's neck, chest and waist.

D Clean casualty's mouth and nose, and remove any dentures, vomit, food or saliva, using a tissue or handkerchief over your fingers.

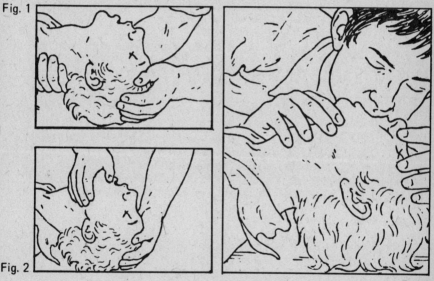

Fig. 1

Fig. 2

Fig. 3

E Place one of your hands under the neck and the other on the forehead so that the casualty's head is tilted backwards (Fig. 1).

F Using the hand from under the neck, lift the chin upwards (Fig. 2); this simple procedure often clears the airway, when the casualty will take a breath and start to breathe on his own. But it is important to keep the head in this position for the clear airway to be maintained until consciousness returns.

G However, if breathing does not start, pinch the casualty's nostrils together, take in a breath yourself, cover casualty's mouth completely and firmly with yours, and breathe into his lungs (Fig. 3).

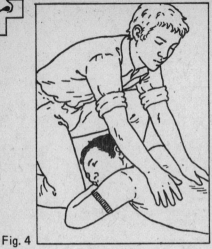
Fig. 4

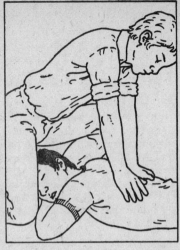
Fig. 5

H From the corner of your eye you will see his chest rise. Remove your mouth and turn your head away, and the chest will fall (casualty breathing out).

I Repeat this procedure rapidly three times, to saturate the casualty's blood with oxygen, then continue the procedure regularly at the rate of about twelve times a minute. To pace yourself, here is a useful gimmick. *In your mind* keep repeating the following jingle at a lively rate:

> '*Turn head, breathe in, turn back,*
> *Breathe out: I've got the knack.*'

J If the chest fails to rise, make sure that the head is tilted well back and the air passages are clear, and start again.

You can continue to give the Kiss of Life until the casualty breathes unaided. If you have been unable to summon help to send for an ambulance earlier, you can now arrange yourself for an ambulance to get the casualty to hospital.

For children and infants, use the same routine, but remember the following points:

A Your mouth may be placed over both mouth and nose of the child.

B Breathe out more gently into the child.

The artificial respiration routine

In certain conditions the Kiss of Life cannot be administered—for example, when the face is damaged or the jaw-bone broken, or if the casualty has swallowed a poison which has burned the lips and mouth. The casualty must then be given artificial respiration.

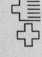

A Send for an ambulance, using any helper for the purpose.

B Place the casualty face downwards with the arms bent so that the casualty's head rests on his hands, with the head turned to one side.

C Kneel on one knee at the casualty's head with the foot of your opposite leg placed near the casualty's elbow.

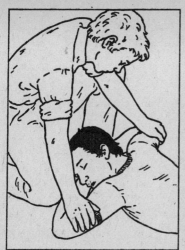

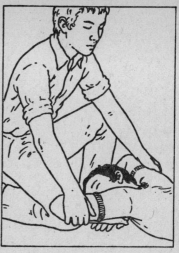

Fig. 6   Fig. 7

D Place your hands on casualty's back just below the shoulder blades or wing bones (Fig. 4).

E Now rock forward with your arms held straight at the elbows until your arms are vertical (upright), at the same time pressing down to compress the chest (Fig. 5).

F At the end of the compression allow your hands to slide sideways and outwards onto casualty's arms just above the elbows (Fig. 6).

G Then rock backwards, lifting casualty's elbows until some resistance is felt at casualty's shoulders (Fig. 7).

H This movement of compression and expansion should last for $2\frac{1}{2}$ seconds and be repeated every five seconds, or twelve times a minute, until casualty starts breathing. To pace yourself, use this slightly different jingle:

'Press down, slide out, pull back
I think I've got the knack.'

For children and infants use the same routine, but using finger tips on the shoulder blades instead of flat hands.

If there was no helper to send for an ambulance earlier, you can now arrange yourself for an ambulance to get the casualty to hospital.

Common causes of failure to breathe

Breathing stops only when there is a definite reason for it to do so. Here are some common causes, with the action you should take.

DROWNING

Clear airway and give Kiss of Life, and perhaps also heart massage or cardiac compression (see pages 43–4 and 46–9).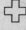

SUFFOCATION BY SMOKE

Remove casualty from smoke area and give Kiss of Life (see pages 43–4). Always bend low in a smoke-filled room.

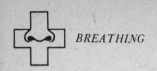

BREATHING

GAS POISONING
Remove casualty from gas into fresh air. Turn off leaking gas and give Kiss of Life (see pages 43–4).

CHOKING
Remove obstruction in airway if possible, giving three or four sharp blows between the shoulder blades. Up-end casualty if possible and continue to strike between the shoulder blades. If breathing stops, give Kiss of Life (see pages 43–4).

ELECTRICITY
Switch off current and give Kiss of Life and heart massage (see pages 43–4 and 46–9).

LIGHTNING
Give Kiss of Life and heart massage (see pages 43–4 and 46–9).

DRUGS
Clear airway and give Kiss of Life (and maybe heart massage) (see pages 43–4 and 46–9).

ACUTE ASTHMA
Asthma is the medical word for a wheezy chest. It is caused by a number of conditions of which the more common are:
1 Infection of the respiratory tract, ie bronchitis.
2 Allergy to pollen, dust, moulds, fur, and other airborne particles.
3 Anxiety and worry.
4 Heart disease.
5 Any combination of 1 to 4.

Treatment
A In the acute attack, allow the casualty to sit up or be propped up with pillows and cushions, in a good clean atmosphere.
B Talk to him quietly and gently to relax him.
C Allow casualty to use inhaler if he has one, according to the dose prescribed.
D Allow casualty to take tablets if he has any, according to the dose prescribed.
E Send for a doctor as soon as possible.
F Do not raise dust by cleaning the room in readiness for the doctor. Do not allow flowers in the room.
G If oxygen is available, and only if you know how to administer it, give oxygen for periods of 5 minutes at a time, until the doctor orders otherwise.

Heart massage (cardiac compression)

46 Life is maintained by the continuing working of the heart and

circulation of the blood. If the heart stops then the body will die; if the circulation fails then the life of the casualty is in danger. You must therefore be able to recognize when the heart has stopped and to do this you must carry out the See, Hear and Feel routine

LOOK AND SEE
1 Blue colour of the face, lips, lobes of ears, fingers and toes.
2 The pupils of the eyes (black part) are widely dilated (enlarged).
3 No pulsation visible in the neck or in the front of the chest.

LISTEN
By placing your ear over the front of the left side of the chest you will normally be able to hear the heart-beat. When the heart has stopped you are unable to hear the heart-beat.

FEEL
1 There should be a pulse in the neck. No pulse can be felt when the heart has stopped.
2 Sometimes the heart-beat can be felt through the chest wall (left front). When the heart has stopped the heart-beat cannot be felt.

If therefore in unconscious casualties you see blueness and dilated pupils, feel no pulsation in the neck or chest, and hear no heart-beat in the chest, you must accept that the heart has stopped and you must start immediate heart massage.

It only takes a few seconds to examine a person to find whether the heart has stopped, so you are not wasting time in carrying out this routine before starting heart massage, more especially because heart massage must *never* be carried out on anyone whose heart has not in fact stopped.

Treatment
A The casualty must be lying on the ground or a hard surface.
B Turn the casualty onto his back, as if looking up to the sky.
C Kneel at one side of the chest (the most convenient side, giving you the most room to move about).
D Find the lower half of the breastbone (the bone to which the ribs are joined in the front of the chest—Fig. 8).

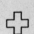

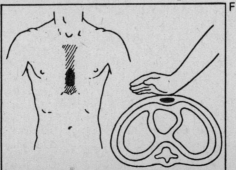

Fig. 8

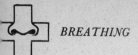

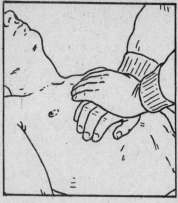

Fig. 9

E Place the heel of the right hand on the lower half of the breastbone.

F Place the left hand on top of the right (Fig. 9).

G With your arms straight push vertically down on the lower half of the breastbone for about 4 cm (1½") in the adult.

H Repeat the pressure between 60–70 times a minute for adults. For children the rate is 80–90 per minute and you push the chest down about 2½ cm (1"). For infants the rate is 90–100 per minute and you push the chest down about 1½ cm (½").

The rhythm of the pressure down should be as regular and even as possible.

If your treatment is being given correctly you will quickly see an improvement in the colour of the casualty, ie the blueness will disappear and the pupils will return to normal size. You will also start to see the pulsations in the neck again. You will be able to hear the heart-beat again in the chest. The See, Hear and Feel routine will tell you that your treatment is successful.

If you happen to be alone with a casualty when his heart and breathing stop, you are still able to carry out heart massage and the Kiss of Life as described, but you have to remember to alternate the giving of each. The rate is fifteen presses to two quick chest inflations (two Kiss of Life).

If you are fortunate enough to have a companion with you, first call an ambulance and then one of you can carry out the Kiss of Life and the other, the heart massage (Fig. 10). The rate then is five presses to one chest inflation.

If the Kiss of Life and heart massage is really working because you and your companion have been carrying out the instructions correctly, a response in the casualty usually occurs within a few minutes of starting the operation, but this does not always follow. It may be necessary to continue the procedure for quite a long time before the casualty responds or the doctor arrives. Once the heart starts to beat again on its own, call an ambulance. You must remain with the casualty until you are able to hand him over to an ambulance attendant or doctor—in case the heart stops again and you have to start the whole process once more.

There are of course a number of people who, despite well

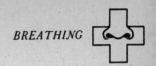

applied Kiss of Life and heart massage will not recover from their heart stopping no matter how long you carry out the procedures, but despite such failures when you are confronted with someone whose heart stops beating you must *try your very best* to get it going again. Only time will prove your efforts to be in vain if the casualty is beyond help—and he may not be.

It is important to remember that if a period of five minutes or more has passed from the time the heart stops to the commencement of the Kiss of Life and heart massage, recovery is unlikely to take place, and the casualty must be considered dead.

Summary of the breathing routines

In an emergency, establish:

A Is the casualty breathing?

B If not, make certain his airway is clear.

C Start the Kiss of Life: 3 quick breaths first, check rise and fall of chest, check colour of casualty.

D Check heart-beat, look at pupils of eyes.

E If no heart-beat, start heart massage.

F The control procedure for one and two helpers is:

No. of helpers	Kiss of Life (No. of breaths)	to	Heart Massage (No. of presses)
1	2		15
2	1		5

The helper on heart massage does the counting, and the helper on Kiss of Life falls into rhythm on the fifth press.

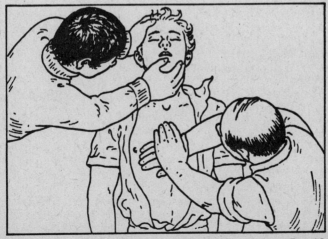

Fig. 10

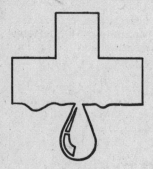

Chapter 5

Bleeding

Bleeding (haemorrhage) is loss of blood from the surface of the body or from any organ within the body. Wherever it occurs, and from whatever cause, every effort must be made to stop it as quickly as possible.

Symptoms of heavy loss of blood

The casualty will exhibit some or all of the following symptoms:
1 Face may be pale.
2 Skin of face, hands and arms may be cold and clammy.
3 Pulse may be rapid and feeble.
4 Breathing may be faster than usual.
5 Pupils of eyes may be dilated.
6 Casualty may faint or pass out.
When a very heavy loss of blood takes place from the surface of the body (in cases of multiple injuries), or internally (from damage to the liver, spleen, kidneys or from the womb in cases of miscarriage, childbirth or very heavy periods), urgent treatment in hospital is required for the patient. A casualty who has lost blood may require a blood transfusion as soon as possible, and this can only be carried out in hospital. You should therefore carry out certain procedures without delay.
A Lay the casualty down (in the Recovery Position if unconscious—see page 34 for Recovery Position routine).
B Raise the feet and legs so that the head remains lower than the body. This allows the blood remaining in the body to be used by the heart, and circulate through the brain thereby supplying it with food and oxygen.
C If the patient happens to be lying on a bed or a stretcher then raise the foot end and place it on one or two chairs or on a coffee table or other low object, so that the whole body is tilted with the head lower than the feet.

D Arrange for the patient to be sent to hospital as quickly as possible.

Surface bleeding

Bleeding from the surface of the body is treated in the following ways.

A Apply pressure with the fingers and/or thumb over the point of bleeding (Fig. 1). Pressure should be maintained for between 5 and 15 minutes.

B When readily available, a dressing may be placed over the wound before pressure is applied (Fig. 2). But if the blood is flowing fast it is best to apply pressure with the thumb or fingers without the dressing.

C If the wound is large then press the edges firmly together with the fingers and thumbs (Fig. 3).

D When possible, apply a clean sterile dressing to the wound, and bandage it tightly enough to apply pressure to the wound, so that it no longer bleeds. Care must be taken here to see that the bandage is not so tight that it completely cuts off the blood supply to other parts of the body. The casualty, if conscious, will usually tell you whether the bandage has been tied too tightly. If so, loosen it a little, but still keep it tight enough to stop bleeding from the wound. Another simple test can be carried out by gently pressing the skin near the wound; this should go white on exerting pressure and quickly go back to pink on release of pressure. If the bandage is too tight, the skin will remain white after release of pressure (Fig. 4).

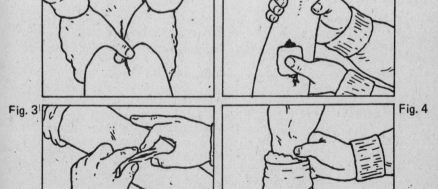

Fig. 1 Fig. 2 Fig. 3 Fig. 4

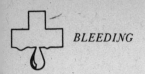

E If a wound on an arm or leg is severe it is advisable to lay the casualty down and raise the leg or arm above the level of the heart, but *not* if there is a fracture or broken bone in the wound.

F If bleeding continues through the dressing and after raising the limb (Fig. 5), then another dressing must be applied on top of the first and bound up tight with another bandage. (On no account should the first dressing be removed.) This should stop the bleeding provided it is tight enough (Fig. 6).

G Where a wound was gaping before you applied a dressing, it most likely will need stitching. In such a case, after applying a suitable dressing and controlling the bleeding, take the casualty to hospital by car or call an ambulance.

Fig. 5

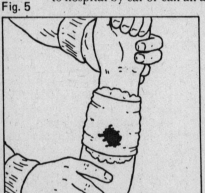 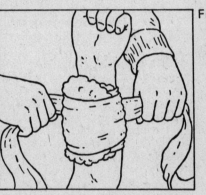

Fig

In major accidents with deep wounds or where limbs are torn off (ie by machinery or carnivorous animals such as wolves, large cats, birds of prey and sharks), there will be heavy blood loss and severe shock.

Treatment

LARGE WOUNDS

A Pack large dressings firmly into the depths of the wound and build up to surface level.

B Bandage firmly to apply pressure over the dressing.

C Elevate if possible.

D Seek medical aid quickly.

TORN-OFF LIMBS

A Initially bleeding should be controlled by a firm pad and bandaging and by elevating the stump, as for large wounds.

B If bleeding continues, apply a constrictive bandage—a crêpe, elastic or other firm bandage may be used, or if none available, a belt or braces. This should be firmly bound around the limb in one place, as close to the stump as possible.

C Every 20 minutes the bandage must be released for 30 seconds.

D Seek medical aid quickly.

E Whenever possible the torn-off limb *must be kept* for surgery.

WHEN THERE IS A FOREIGN BODY IN THE WOUND

This may be, for instance, a piece of glass, wood or metal.

A Apply pressure with your fingers or thumbs along the edge of the wound, leaving the foreign body in its place inside the wound (Fig. 7). *Do not* remove the foreign body.

B Apply dressings along the edge of the wound and hold them in place with a tight bandage, still leaving the foreign body in place (Fig. 8).

C If the wound is in an arm or leg and the bleeding profuse, lay the casualty down and raise the arm or leg above the level of the heart.

D Arrange for an ambulance. or take the casualty to hospital by car.

Bleeding from within the body

This can take several forms, and these are explained below.

BLEEDING NOSE

This is a common occurrence in the younger age groups, usually due to a small blood vessel breaking and bleeding, just inside one or other nostril. Nose-bleeding is usually brought about by bangs on the nose, rubbing it excessively or through picking. It does not normally bleed for very long if the following treatment is carried out.

Treatment

A Sit the casualty down.

B Tilt the head slightly forward.

C Allow the blood to drip from the nose into a bowl or basin.

D Pinch the soft part of the nose (Fig. 9).

E Tell the casualty to avoid swallowing blood.

F Bleeding usually stops within a few minutes. Casualty should rest after treatment for at least one hour. In repeated nose bleeds of this nature the casualty should seek the advice of his doctor.

Nose bleeding in older age groups is often due to a raised blood pressure, and is frequently considered a safety valve in such cases.

Fig. 7

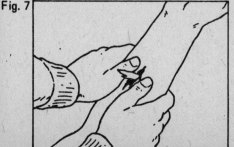

Fig. 8

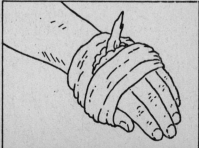

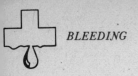
Treatment

Carry out the same procedure as for younger age groups, but if bleeding does not stop in a matter of minutes and continues at a steady drip, the advice of a doctor should be sought at once. Do not plug the nose.

COUGHING BLOOD IN QUANTITY FROM THE LUNGS

Coughing blood in quantity (ie a small cupful or more) is not a common occurrence but when it does occur it is very frightening for·both the patient and relatives. It is usually the result of a disease of the lungs, such as a lung cancer or severe tuberculosis, or some form of perforating injury to the lungs.

Treatment

Fig. 9

A Lay the casualty down with the head and shoulders slightly raised and inclined towards the injured side (Fig. 10).

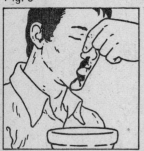
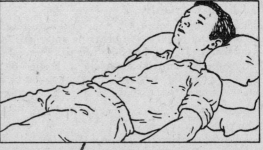

Fig. 10

B Do not give any food or liquid by mouth.
C If bleeding from the lungs is caused by a wound to the chest, then a firm padded dressing covered with a piece of polythene must be applied over the wound and secured as firmly as possible, to prevent air being sucked into the wound and so into the chest cavity, thereby causing other possible complications (Figs. 11, 12 and 13).
D Send for your doctor immediately or arrange for an ambulance to take the casualty to hospital.

Fig. 11

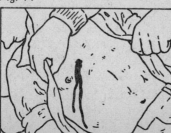
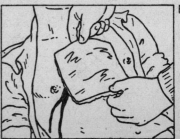

Fig. 12

54

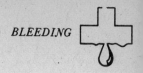

VOMITING BLOOD FROM THE STOMACH

This is usually due to a stomach ulcer that has been bleeding. When the stomach has filled with blood, it suddenly contracts and the casualty vomits up all the blood and this may amount to as much as a litre or more.

Treatment

A Lay the casualty down with the feet and legs raised higher than the body.

B Keep the casualty at a reasonable temperature. Do not over-heat by applying too many blankets or hot water bottles—keep the casualty just warm, and do not let him shiver with cold.

C Do not give any food or liquid by mouth.

D The mouth may be washed out with water, but none must be swallowed.

E Send immediately for a doctor, or arrange for an ambulance to take the casualty to hospital.

F If the casualty becomes unconscious, he must immediately be turned on his side in the Recovery Position (Fig. 14), but still keeping the feet and legs raised. For Recovery Position routine, see page 34.

HEAVY BLEEDING FROM THE WOMB (uterus)

This may occur in women from puberty when periods first start until they stop at the change of life, or menopause; only occasionally does it occur after that time, but it can do so and be a heavy loss. The usual causes of heavy bleeding are:

1 A heavy period which may contain clots.
2 The result of a miscarriage or abortion.
3 During pregnancy.
4 During or immediately after childbirth.
5 After a 'D & C' treatment (scraping of the womb)—usually within a few days.

Treatment

A Lay the patient down with the feet and legs raised above the level of the chest.

B Keep the casualty at a reasonable temperature. Do not over-heat by applying too many blankets or hot water bottles.

C Do not give any food or liquid by mouth.

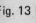
Fig. 13

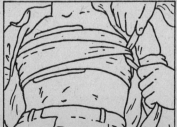

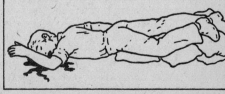

Fig. 14

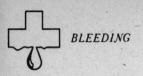

 D Send immediately for a doctor or arrange for ambulance to take the casualty to hospital.

E Whilst waiting place some thick towelling under the patient and between the legs.

BLEEDING FROM THE BACK PASSAGE

Anal or rectal bleeding may be dark, black and sticky, showing that the blood has come from high up in the bowel and has been altered during its passage down the bowel. The patient may show symptoms of shock and feel very ill.

Treatment

A Lay the patient down with the feet and legs raised above the level of the chest.

B Keep the casualty at a reasonable temperature. Do not over-heat by applying too many blankets or hot water bottles.

C Do not give any food or liquids by mouth.

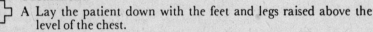 D Send immediately for a doctor or arrange for an ambulance to take the patient to hospital.

Bleeding from the back passage which is bright red in colour often occurs from piles (haemorrhoids). It is rarely severe and stops quickly after the bowels have been opened. In these cases the best thing is for the patient to see his own doctor. The bleeding may, however, be heavy and severe, causing the patient to show signs of severe loss of blood.

Treatment

A Lay the patient down with the feet and legs raised above the level of the chest.

B Keep the casualty at a reasonable temperature. Do not over-heat by applying too many blankets or hot water bottles.

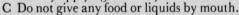 C Send immediately for a doctor or arrange for an ambulance to take the patient to hospital.

D Whilst waiting place some thick towelling under the buttocks of the casualty and apply a cold dressing to the piles.

SUSPECTED BLEEDING FROM THE LIVER, SPLEEN OR KIDNEYS

Bleeding from one or other of these organs occurs from:

1 Violent blunt blow over the abdomen, the right upper side for the liver, the left upper side for the spleen, or the loins for either kidney. Such injury may result, for example, from kicks from horses, heavy objects falling onto the abdomen, punches in the loins, or the wheel of a vehicle passing over the abdomen.

2 Stab wounds, bullet wounds or any other penetrating object in the areas described will produce severe bleeding internally in the abdomen.

3 Disease.

To diagnose this type of bleeding you must carry out the See, Hear and Feel routine.

See

A Look for the object that may have caused the injury.
B Look for bruising of the abdominal wall.
C Look at the colour of the face—pale.
D See how ill the casualty appears to be.
E The rate of respiration will be much faster than usual—about 24 per minute or more. Shallow type.
F Look for dilation of pupils of the eyes.

Hear

A Ask what happened if the patient is conscious.
B Ask where the pain is.
C Ask if mouth is dry.
D Ask if there is any history of an injury to any of the places marked X in Fig. 15.

Fig. 15

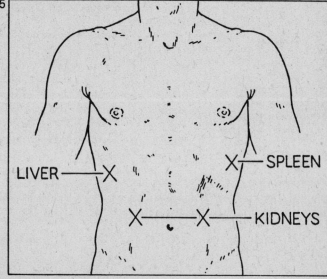

Feel

A Take the pulse rate at the wrist—usually in the range of 110 or above, feeble, rapid.
B Feel the cold clammy skin of the face, hands and arms.
C Feel gently the abdomen—patient will feel the pain made worse as you press over the liver or spleen or kidneys.
D Take the pulse again and you may well find it faster than the first time you took it

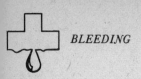

BLEEDING

Treatment

A Lay the casualty down (in the Recovery Position if unconscious—see page 34 for Recovery Position routine).

B Raise the feet, legs and trunk so that the head is lower than the rest of the body.

C Despite thirst, give nothing by mouth. Casualty may be allowed to rinse mouth, but swallow nothing.

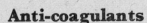

D Arrange for the casualty to go to hospital as quickly as possible.

Anti-coagulants

Many convalescents returning from hospital have been given tablets to prevent their blood from clotting, especially those who have been treated for coronary thrombosis or thrombosis of a deep vein in the leg. Such patients are advised to have their blood checked at regular intervals in order to adjust the dose of anti-coagulant tablets. This is important, as too big a dose may cause even the smallest and simplest of wounds to bleed. It is necessary, therefore, for the following signs and symptoms to be noted and acted upon immediately they develop.

1 Bleeding continuing from a simple wound which cannot be stopped by direct pressure for five minutes.

2 Bleeding from the nose persisting after simple measures to stop it have been taken.

3 Bleeding from the bowel.

4 Blood in the urine.

5 Blood in phlegm coughed up from chest.

6 Vomiting of blood.

7 Swelling of a knee or other joint following a simple blow.

8 Sudden onset of partial or complete blindness.

Treatment

A Should any of these symptoms develop, you or the casualty must immediately contact the hospital controlling the anti-coagulant dosage.

B Bleeding must be controlled (see pages 50–1) until advice is obtained.

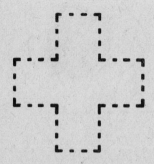

Chapter 6

Unconsciousness

The loss of consciousness is always a serious sign. Unconsciousness is described as the state in which the human being will not respond in any way to shaking, shouting or pinching. If a person who appears unconscious recovers and 'comes to' quickly when shaken, spoken to sharply, or pinched—and instantly knows where he is and who he is—then that person was asleep and not unconscious.

In casualties who are only just unconscious, the eyes may be moving about and when a bright light is shone into them the pupils contract. In people who are deeply unconscious, however, the eyes may be fixed as if looking straight ahead with the pupils dilated (bigger than normal); the pupils will not contract when a light is shone into them. In these conditions—with the pupils dilated and the eyes fixed in one position—it usually means that the casualty is near to death. When you find a person apparently unconscious, apply the Shake, Shout and Pinch routine. If there is no response, he is unconscious.

Treatment

A Place the casualty in the Recovery Position in the following manner: turn him onto his back.

B Tuck his left arm under the left buttock (Fig. 1).

C Place the right arm above the head (Fig. 1).

Fig. 1

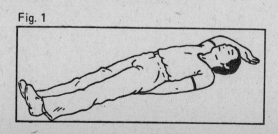

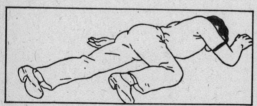

Fig. 2

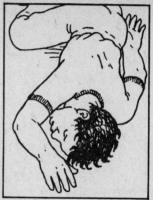

Fig.

D Pull the body over on top of the left side.

E Bend the right leg up to the bent position.

F Bend the right arm into the bent position (Fig. 2).

G Clear away anything loose from the mouth and throat, including dentures, thus producing a clear airway so that casualty may breathe easily.

H Ease the left arm out behind the body.

I Now lift the head upwards and backwards to ensure that the airway is clear (Fig. 3).

This is the left-side Recovery Position, but it may be more convenient to turn the casualty into the right-side Recovery Position, in which case carry out the above routine substituting right for left and vice versa.

In cases where it is impossible to turn the casualty into the Recovery Position owing to the presence of other injuries, or his being trapped, then the maintenance of a clear airway is carried out by placing two fingers behind the angle of the jaw on both sides and pushing the jaw forward towards the nose. This will force the tongue forward and away from the back of the throat, so clearing the airway. If this simple procedure should fail to clear the airway, then open the mouth, clear any debris from it and then hold the tongue between the folds of a handkerchief and pull it forwards. The airway should then be clear.

It is important to remember that the airway must be *kept* clear in one of these ways until it is automatically kept clear by placing the casualty in the Recovery Position or until a doctor or other trained person has passed a special type of breathing tube. But only a doctor or trained person can pass such a tube. The untrained person attempting to pass a tube may do more harm than good to the casualty.

J Do not give any food or liquid by mouth, as this will make the casualty choke and block the airway so that he cannot breathe.

K Send for a doctor or call for an ambulance to take the casualty to hospital.

L Whilst awaiting the arrival of the doctor or ambulance you must not only maintain the clear airway, but treat any other injuries the casualty may have sustained.

If the casualty appears dead, ie if the breathing and heart appear to have just stopped, then the Kiss of Life and heart massage must be started immediately. A doctor or ambulance must also be summoned as soon as possible.

If the casualty is stiff from having died some time previously then leave the casualty in the position in which you find him and call a doctor and, where appropriate, the police.

Causes of unconsciousness

There is an opportunity, while waiting for the doctor or ambulance to arrive, to try and discover the cause of unconsciousness. The common causes of unconsciousness are:
Fainting
Head injury
Stroke
Epilepsy—major fits or convulsions
Minor fits
Heart attacks
Diabetes
Drugs
Drink
Severe bleeding
Acute and severe allergy
Electric shock
Drowning
Gas poisoning.

THE COMMON FAINT

This occurs often in children and less frequently in adults, when they stand in one position for a long time, especially if they are not well or during very hot weather; or when they have had no food or liquids for several hours. When a person is going to faint he goes quite pale or white, with beads of perspiration on the forehead. The skin becomes cold and clammy, and he may feel he is going to be sick. Then he gently falls to the ground in a heap. If the pulse is taken at the wrist, it is usually very fast and quite weak to feel.

Provided the casualty is in no further danger, as from fire or traffic, turn him into the Recovery Position when you will find that he will rapidly recover, in a matter of five to ten minutes. After a further short period of three to five minutes it is safe to allow him to sit up and take a glass of cold water, and then, a little later on, a cup of sweet tea. If he is feeling quite normal after a rest of fifteen minutes, he may return to whatever he was originally doing. In cases of lack of food and liquids, a strong cup of sweet tea with milk and a biscuit will be helpful. This, together with a period of rest, should produce a full and normal recovery.

HEAD INJURY

In such cases it should be obvious that the casualty has received a blow to the skull, as for example, a car driver hitting the windscreen, a motor cyclist thrown off his motor cycle, a rider falling off his horse, a housewife falling off a ladder or down stairs. The clues are:

1 A wound is usually seen on the skull, with bleeding occurring— often quite profuse. The casualty will look pale and shocked. Pulse rate will be 90 or more in the adult.
2 The casualty will have fallen into an odd position, the airway will be restricted and therefore the breathing will be noisy.
3 Occasionally there is slight bleeding or fluid leaking from the the ear or nose.
4 One pupil may be bigger than the other, with neither contracting when a light is shone into the eyes.
5 There may be bloodstained froth at the mouth.
6 The casualty may go into a convulsion (a fit) while still unconscious.

Treatment

A Carefully supporting the head, turn the casualty into the Recovery Position.
B Place a loose dressing or handkerchief under the ear (unattached) so that a doctor may assess the nature of the fluid loss.
C Control bleeding from any wound that can be seen by direct pressure and by the use of appropriate dressings and bandages. This does not apply to leakage from the ear.
D Keep casualty in the Recovery Position and keep the airway clear.
E Do not leave the casualty while he is unconscious.
F Do not give any food or liquids by mouth.
G Send for a doctor or call for an ambulance.

STROKE

This usually occurs in the middle-aged to elderly, but can in rare cases occur in the young. It is due to bleeding from a burst blood vessel inside or on the surface of the brain. It is of sudden onset and usually without any warning to the patient. If there is warning the casualty complains of a severe headache, gradually getting worse, followed by sudden collapse. The clues are:

1 Casualty often looks pale and shocked, but sometimes the face can be flushed with a purple colour.
2 The lips may be blue.
3 One side of the face may blow out with each breath whilst the opposite side remains tense: breathing will be noisy.
4 Frothing at the nose and mouth from saliva.
5 The casualty will be limp down one side of the body whilst the the opposite side will be tense.

6 The pupils may be of different sizes and will not react to light; alternatively, they may be equal in size and dilated.
7 The casualty may well pass urine or even have his bowels open.
8 The casualty may have a convulsion.
9 There may be twitching of the muscles of the face and limbs.
10 The pulse at the wrist may be rapid and very forceful. It is easily felt.

Treatment

A Immediately turn the casualty into the Recovery Position (see page 34).
B Make quite sure the airway is clear.
C Loosen tight clothing.
D Send for a doctor or call for an ambulance.
E Clean up casualty after urination or bowel action.

EPILEPSY, CONVULSIONS OR FITS

These conditions *(grand mal)* can occur in any age group. It is fairly common in infancy, brought about by high temperature which in turn is frequently due to a throat or chest infection. But any infection of an infant causing a high temperature can be the underlying cause of an infantile convulsion.

In older children and adults suffering fits the common cause is unknown. In these cases it is important to remember that the casualty often has no indication he is going to suffer a fit. Instead he suddenly falls to the ground and convulses. During the convulsion, the casualty throws his arms and legs in all directions with no control, grits his teeth tightly and froths at the mouth. He goes purple in the face and usually passes urine. The convulsion lasts approximately 45 seconds but may vary in length from individual to individual ie 30 seconds to 90 seconds, or even longer.

Treatment: infantile convulsion

A During the actual fit control the child so that it does no harm to itself by hitting hard or sharp objects.
B Once the fit is over, turn the child into the Recovery Position (see page 34) and sponge him down with lukewarm water (*not* ice cold).
C Once the temperature has been reduced, cuddle the child and allow him to sleep, always making sure that the airway is kept clear.
D Send for a doctor.
E The infant usually recovers from such an attack during the following half hour to one hour. Continue to sponge the child down with lukewarm water to keep the body below the temperature that caused the convulsion.

Treatment: the older child or adult

A During the actual convulsion all that can be done is to prevent the casualty doing damage to himself whilst throwing his arms and legs about, eg preventing an arm or leg from going into an open fire, through a greenhouse window, or into a piece of moving machinery.

B Immediately the convulsion is over the casualty should be turned into the Recovery Position (see page 34), the mouth opened and cleaned of froth and saliva, and any dentures removed.

C Loosen all tight clothing around the neck, chest and waist, ie, tie, bra, corsets, belt, elastics and trousers.

D After the convulsion is over, the casualty relaxes and usually goes into a deep sleep. Provided he is in the Recovery Position he will come to no harm. After half an hour or more, he usually awakens and complains of headache, muscle aches and complete exhaustion. Allow the casualty to rest for the whole day.

E If the convulsion happens to be the first that the casualty has ever suffered, then a doctor must be sent for or he must be admitted to hospital immediately. If however the casualty is known to suffer from epileptic fits, then seek guidance from his relatives or those who know him well, as to whether a doctor is required, or whether the casualty should go to hospital.

MINOR FITS

These fits are short periods of blankness occurring in children or young adults only. They last for a few seconds only. One fit may occur on its own to be followed by another some hours later, but more often they occur at intervals of a minute and last about 5 to 10 seconds. They are most often recognized when a child is asked a question and an immediate answer is not given. The recognition of these fits is often done at school by the teachers. It is thought at first to be stupidity or bad manners, but if the child is observed he will be seen to have these short periods of blankness which he cannot help. No treatment is necessary at the time that the child suffers the attacks, but the child must be taken to a doctor for long-term treatment.

HEART ATTACKS

The commonest sudden heart attack is due to an obstruction of one of the coronary arteries that supply the heart muscle with blood and thus with oxygen and food substances. When a coronary artery blocks off, the muscle beyond the blockage does not receive a blood supply containing oxygen and food. The muscle therefore fails and in consequence the heart as a whole may fail and possibly stop altogether.

The casualty suffering a coronary thrombosis usually complains of a severe tight pain across the upper chest, like a tight band round the chest continually being tightened. The pain often spreads up the front of the neck, and down the inside of the left arm; occasionally it may spread down the inside of the right arm.

If the pain gets too great and the heart fails to survive, the blood supply to the brain begins to fail and the casualty then becomes unconscious. The pulse is usually rapid and tends to be feeble and as the attack progresses the fingers may become blue, and finally the pupils of the eye dilate. The position in which the casualty falls will decide whether the airway will block. Vomiting often occurs, and this also tends to block the airway.

Treatment

A If the casualty is sitting comfortably and is conscious then leave him sitting still and send for a doctor.

B If the casualty collapses to the floor and becomes unconscious, turn him into the Recovery Position (see page 34).

C Clear the airway.

D Constantly check that the heart is beating.

E If the heart stops, start heart massage (see pages 46–9).

F Send for a doctor or call for an ambulance.

DIABETES

Diabetes is a medical condition in which the quantity of sugar in the blood rises above a certain level. In this condition a person can become unconscious, and this applies also if the quantity of sugar in the blood falls below a certain level.

In all humans the state of consciousness depends on the blood containing the correct quantity of sugar in solution. In the untreated diabetic the quantity of sugar in the blood rises over a period of time (days or weeks) and when it reaches too high a level the person becomes unconscious.

In the treated diabetic patient, taking injections of insulin, another type of unconsciousness or coma can occur. Insulin works in the body by reducing the amount of sugar circulating in the blood. If it reduces the sugar quantity too quickly or by too much, the casualty quite suddenly becomes unconscious, usually with only a short warning of a few minutes or even seconds. During this period the casualty may have slurred speech, be irritable and obstructive. A careful search of the casualty may reveal a card or medic-alert bracelet, confirming your diagnosis of diabetes. Once unconscious, he goes deeper into coma until appropriate treatment is given by a doctor.

Treatment

A During the period of slurred speech or irritability, sugar may be given by mouth, but once the casualty becomes unconscious *nothing* should be given by mouth, and a doctor should be called, or the casualty sent to hospital.

B Once the casualty has become unconscious he must be turned into the Recovery Position (see page 34) and the airway cleared of any obstruction.

C Do not leave the casualty while he is unconscious.

DRUGS

A large proportion of drugs and medicines when taken in too great a quantity at one time will produce a state of unconsciousness. This applies equally to drugs prescribed by a doctor or obtained through a drug pusher.

Treatment (unconscious)

A Turn casualty into the Recovery Position (see page 34).

B Clear his airway.

C Call for a doctor and ambulance.

D A close watch must be kept on breathing and heartbeat. If either or both fail, the Kiss of Life and/or heart massage must be started immediately (see pages 43–4 and 46–9).

E Do not remove or destroy the empty bottles in which the tablets or medicine were contained, and do not remove any vomit from around the casualty. The bottles and specimens of vomit should be sent to the hospital for testing in the laboratory.

F If the person is obviously dead, then you must also send for the police and not touch anything in the room where the person is lying.

Treatment (conscious)

A If the casualty has taken a large quantity of drugs and is still conscious, then you must endeavour to keep him conscious by talking to him.

B Arrange for urgent admission to hospital.

C Again the empty bottles or any vomit must be kept for analysis.

D Do not give large quantities of fluid such as water or an emetic; and do not make the casualty vomit to get rid of the drugs. It is safer and better to get a doctor or get the casualty to hospital in as short a time as possible.

DRINK

Alcohol is a poison and if taken in sufficiently large quantities may result in death. Anyone who has reached the stage where it is difficult to walk or speak may become unconscious and may vomit (in that order); it is therefore essential to place the casualty in the Recovery Position and keep the airway clear. Where a casualty is found unconscious, the smell of alcohol on the breath does not necessarily mean that the casualty is intoxicated. The amount of alcohol consumed cannot be assessed, and the casualty may only have taken a sip of brandy because he felt unwell. It is essential therefore to examine unconscious casualties for other injuries.

Treatment
A Place casualty in the Recovery Position (see page 34).
B Loosen clothing at neck and waist.
C Examine casualty for other injuries.
D Seek medical aid or get casualty to hospital by ambulance.

SEVERE BLEEDING
In very severe bleeding a casualty may become unconscious due
to lack of blood reaching the brain, which then lacks oxygen and
necessary food substances. The more common causes of severe
bleeding include: the rupture of one or more of the bigger blood
vessels in the body, eg in the chest or abdomen; bleeding from the
spleen or liver following a blow to the abdomen; disease of the
stomach or bowel; bleeding from the womb at the time of miscarriage or abortion, during or after childbirth, and occasionally
at the time of a very heavy period.

Treatment
In these cases it is usually impossible to apply pressure at the
point where the bleeding is occurring and so stop the loss. When
the casualty is unconscious:
A Place casualty in the Recovery Position (see page 34).
B Clear the airway.
C Raise the legs so that the head is lower than the heart. By this
   means gravity helps as much blood as possible to pass through
   the brain.
D Send for a doctor or ambulance immediately.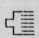

ACUTE ALLERGY
Some people are extra sensitive to wasp or bee stings and when
stung will rapidly become unconscious. Remember that a sting
in the mouth may lead to dangerous swelling.

Treatment
A Place the casualty in the Recovery Position (see page 34).
B Clear the airway.
C Send for a doctor or call for an ambulance immediately.
D Do not leave casualty.
E The maintenance of a clear airway is sometimes difficult to
   achieve due to swelling that occurs in the mouth and throat. If
   there is any tendency for this to occur *before* the casualty
   becomes unconscious, take or send him to hospital where
   breathing apparatus will be provided.

ELECTRIC SHOCK
This is usually easy to identify as the casualty will be lying unconscious near an electrical appliance or cable.

Treatment

A Before touching the casualty remember to switch off the electrical supply.

B If the casualty is breathing, turn him into the Recovery Position (see page 34).

C If the casualty has stopped breathing, you must start the Kiss of Life and heart massage immediately (see pages 43–4 and 46–9).

D Send for a doctor or ambulance.

DROWNING
Treatment

A Clear the airway and determine whether casualty is breathing and the heart pumping.

B If the heart and breathing have stopped, then you immediately start the Kiss of Life and heart massage (see pages 43–4 and 46–9).

C If the casualty is just unconscious, then once removed from the water, he should be placed in the Recovery Position (see page 34).

D A doctor or an ambulance should be sent for immediately.

GAS POISONING
Treatment

A In all cases of unconsciousness from any source of gas, remove the casualty from the affected area and turn off the gas where possible.

B If breathing and heart have stopped, immediately start the Kiss of Life and heart massage (see pages 43–4 and 46–9).

C If the casualty is breathing, but just conscious, then turn him into the Recovery Position (see page 34) and clear the airway.

D Send for a doctor or call for an ambulance immediately.

E If the casualty is obviously dead then the police must be informed.

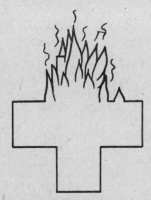

Chapter 7

Burns and scalds

Burns and scalds can have distressing effects, such as scarring, deformity and mental trauma; these effects can all be long-lasting, and sometimes even permanent. Correct, careful and prompt treatment of deep burns is therefore essential.

Burns occur when the body is in contact with, or too close to, dry heat and strong chemicals, and among the many frequent causes are:

1 Kitchen utensils, such as baking tins, oven shelves and pan handles.
2 Modern electrical equipment, including kettles, hotplates and irons.
3 Accidental fires from open grates, gas and electric fires.
4 Clothing and other articles accidentally set alight (Fig. 1).
5 Bleach and undiluted disinfectants.
6 Excessive sun and wind.
7 Accidents with ropes.

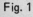 Fig. 1

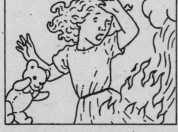 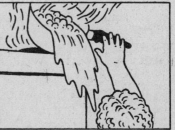 Fig. 2

Because of their character, burns are most often sustained by the exposed parts of the body, particularly the hands, wrists and head. Scalds, on the other hand, occur when the body is in contact with moist heat, such as steam or hot water, fats or oils, and other hot liquids (Fig. 2). But there the difference ends for our purposes, because the resulting effect on the skin is much the same.

In this chapter a 'burn' means a burn or a scald. The damage from burns can range from a mere reddening of the affected skin to blister formation and, in more serious cases, to actual destruction of the tissues. In hospital language, burns are described as being superficial or deep, depending on the depth of the damage. Superficial burns are in fact the more painful. But in first aid it is not the depth, but the surface area of the burn, by which its seriousness is measured.

Most burns happen in the home, so that is where they have to be treated; and as most home accidents take place in the kitchen, the kitchen is probably the best room in which to treat casualties. But here again, we stress the need to avoid accidents, for so many of them need never happen. You cannot read Chapter 1 of *Help!* too often! Remember that the groups at the greatest risk are the elderly, the physically handicapped, and children—especially toddlers. All burns to children and the elderly must be taken seriously.

Some important don'ts

Before describing what burns do to the body and what you can do to help before professional aid is available, here are a few things you must *not* do when these injuries occur.
1 Never put butter, flour or baking soda on a burn.
2 Never use ointments, lotions or oil as treatment.
3 Never prick or break any blisters that may form.
4 Never handle or touch the injury more than absolutely necessary.
5 Never pull away burnt clothing stuck to the body.
Most clothing nowadays is made from synthetic fibres which melt like toffee and stick to the skin. If you attempt to remove it you will tear the skin causing unnecessary pain and inviting infection in. The burnt clothing will have been made sterile and is best left alone.

General treatment

Apart from a few special types of burns (dealt with later in this chapter), there is a common treatment for all the others. Start off by appreciating that burns, other than very small ones, are dangerous, painful and cause shock. Often they are sustained in an emergency, such as a house fire or road accident with a petrol fire. The prime rules of the Help Routine are therefore doubly important and you must remember to keep calm and encourage the casualty, who will be shocked and frightened—be gentle with him—and act quickly yet systematically, always doing first things first.

Once the skin and tissues are burnt, a serious loss of fluid may occur. The affected tissues will hold the heat, and cause further damage and pain. The object of early treatment therefore is to *get rid of the heat*. First aid treatment must reduce the temperature in the damaged tissue.

Treatment

A Immerse the injured part in cold water. This may be done  using a bucket or washing-up bowl, the kitchen sink, or simply holding the burn under a gently running cold tap (Fig. 3). The burn should be immersed in cold water for about fifteen minutes or until the pain has stopped. If it is difficult to immerse the injury (on the face, for instance), soak a clean tea-cloth or any other clean soft material in cold water and apply it to the injury as a compress (Fig. 4). Remember to change the compress repeatedly (by re-soaking in cold water), but do not rub the surface of the burn. This treatment will take some of the heat out of the tissues and prevent further damage, reddening, blistering and pain.

Fig. 3

Fig. 5

Fig. 4

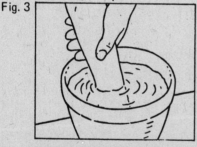

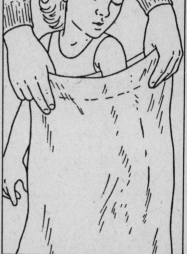

B Remove rings, bracelets, shoes and tight-fitting articles as soon as possible after injury, as swelling may develop making it difficult to remove them later.

C Small superficial burns should be carefully patted dry once pain has stopped, and then covered with a dressing. Larger areas or deep burns when removed from the water should be covered lightly with clean, recently-laundered, non-fluffy material. (A clean pillowcase is ideal for limbs—Fig. 5.)

D Send for a doctor or call for an ambulance.

E Any burn larger than a postage stamp ($2 \times 2\frac{1}{2}$ cm) must be seen by a doctor, who should be summoned *after* you have applied cooling treatment.

F When a large area is damaged, requiring hospital care, ice may be packed in a towel and applied to the injury during the journey.

G It is essential to cover up burnt tissue to prevent infection, which thrives on burnt skin. This also reduces the anxiety of the casualty, who can no longer see the burn. Tablecloths or sheets (*not* nylon) are excellent for covering the body. The covering should be held in place *lightly*.

H While waiting for doctor or ambulance, reassure and comfort casualty. Pick up a child and cuddle: this is most important, but be careful not to do damage in the process.

SUMMARY OF GENERAL TREATMENT

A Flood or immerse burned part in cold water for at least fifteen minutes.

B Remove rings and bracelets.

C Pat dry and cover.

D Send for doctor or ambulance, depending on severity.

Circumstances requiring special treatments

CLOTHES ON FIRE

A If clothing is still on fire, extinguish flames by dowsing with water, or cut off the air supply by wrapping casualty in a blanket, coat or other large piece of material—even a rug. Remember to hold the blanket in front of you to protect you from the flames you are smothering (Fig. 6)!

Fig. 6

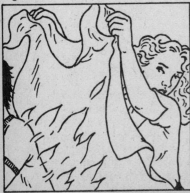

Fig. 7

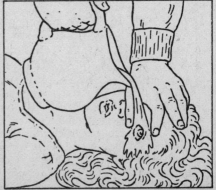

B Anyone on fire is terrified, and may rush from room to room, spreading the fire, or may run into the fresh air where the fire will burn more readily. Therefore encourage the patient to stay still.

C. Once the flames are extinguished continue the general treatment for burns already outlined above.

SUNBURN

This is a burn in the correct sense of the word.

A Remove casualty into the shade.

B Cool affected surface areas as in the general treatment (see pages 70–2).

In severe cases give frequent cold drinks (non-alcoholic).

D Call a doctor.

E Continue the general treatment for burns.

WIND BURNS

The skin can be affected by exposure to high winds.

A Apply moisture cream liberally.

B Cover the exposed area and protect from the wind.

ROPE OR FRICTION BURNS

The burns, usually caused by rope running through the hands or between the legs in gymnastics, sailing or climbing, can be as painful and potentially dangerous as burns from direct heat.

A Cool affected area by placing in cold water.

B When pain has abated, dry gently and cover with a dry dressing.

C If hands must be used, protect affected surfaces with gloves.

CHEMICAL BURNS

As long as the chemical is in contact with the skin it will continue to cause damage. The aim of the treatment is therefore to remove the chemical as quickly as possible.

A Contaminated clothing should be carefully removed and soaked in water. Take care that you do not contaminate yourself.

B Flood the affected area with cold water, washing thoroughly and systematically for ten to fifteen minutes.

C Continue general treatment for burns (see pages 70–2).

CHEMICAL SPLASHES IN THE EYE

This can cause permanent damage and even loss of vision, and therefore *great speed* is required in carrying out the treatment. The chemical must be diluted instantly.

A Lay the casualty on his back and, holding the eyelids apart with thumb and forefinger, pour cold water continuously over the front of the eye from the nose side (to prevent the chemical affecting the other eye—Fig. 7).

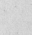

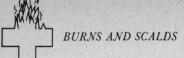

B Allow the eyelids to close and open several times to ensure that no chemical is tucked away in the folds of the lids.

C Continue this washing process for at least ten minutes. Do this by the clock, and *don't cut it short.*

D After treatment, close the lids, place a pad over the eye, and secure lightly in position.

E Comfort casualty and call for an ambulance or take him to hospital.

ELECTRICAL BURNS

These are often quite small in area, but they may nevertheless be quite deep. They are normally found at the points of contact where the current entered and left the body.

A Switch off the current and remove the plug before treating casualty.

B If the casualty is lying in water, keep out of it yourself—moisture is an excellent conductor of electricity. For the same reason do not hold the casualty under the armpits.

C Check the casualty's breathing. The current may have passed through the chest, stopping the heart and stopping breathing. If so start the Kiss of Life and heart massage immediately (see pages 43–4 and 46–9).

D Continue the general treatment for burns (see pages 70–2).

Chapter 8

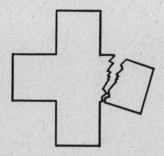

Bones and muscles

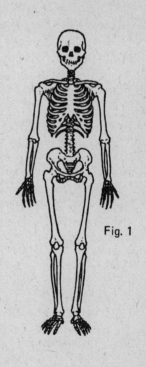

In the human body, under the skin and soft tissues, there are 206 bones of various shapes and sizes, and this framework is called the skeleton (Fig. 1). Wherever two or more bones meet, there is a joint; some joints are intentionally moveable, but many of them are fixed. Those that move can rotate, as at the shoulder or wrist, or they may hinge, as at the elbow and knee. All such movements are natural and healthy. We can make the bones at moveable joints 'waggle' in order to perform their allotted functions.

Examine your body in a long mirror and you will instantly recognize the moveable joints: these, in simple language, are the fingers and toes, wrists and heels, elbows and knees, shoulders and hips, backbone, neck and jawbone. With this in mind, you will not find it difficult to spot unnatural movements. For example, an arm that waggles between the shoulder and elbow can safely be assumed to be broken. Or again, a leg that waggles between the knee and ankle can be assumed to be broken.

Fig. 1

Here we are dealing with injuries to the bones *and* the tissues that surround them. These injuries take the form of broken bones (fractures), torn ligaments (sprains), pulled muscles (strains), and separated joints (dislocations). All are associated in greater or lesser degree with violence in some form, and when they occur,

the first thing to establish is the cause. This can be very important in assisting diagnosis. So:
A Ask what happened.
B Look around for evidence of the accident.
It is a golden rule that if a broken bone is suspected, you should play safe and treat as a fracture.

Diagnosis of fractures

There are a number of important clues that will be present with a broken bone, and the early diagnosis should be developed from a study of these clues.

PAIN

This will always be present, less in small bones, but very intense in large ones.

SHOCK

This is surgical shock brought on by pain and loss of blood. With large fractures the shock will be severe. The clues you are looking for are pale face and fast but feeble pulse.

LOSS OF POWER

The normal use of the broken bone will be restricted, and it may be entirely isolated by sheer pain. At the worst it will be impossible to use it—with a broken leg, standing will usually be impossible. Ask the casualty about this.

SWELLING

In almost all cases there will be swelling of the surrounding tissues. This is because the blow causing the bone to break will also bruise or damage these tissues, and there can also be some bleeding from the bone itself. (In large bones like the thighbone, this bleeding can amount to 1–2 litres (1¾ to 3½ pints), causing very extensive swelling and bruising.)

UNUSUAL SHAPE AND MOVEMENT

The limb, or part of the body having the bone broken, may look odd and misshapen (Fig. 2), and you may feel irregular bumps along the usually smooth surface area. And those 'waggles' between the joints may be noticed.

A broken bone may be the main injury, but equally it may be just part of more serious multiple injuries. Fractures are classified in two groups to determine the treatment the fracture itself should receive at this early stage.

Closed fracture. Here there is damage to the bone, but no break in the skin.

Open fracture. Again the bone is damaged, but this time there is a

Fig. 2

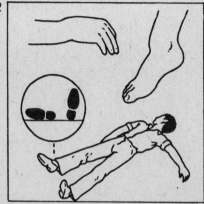
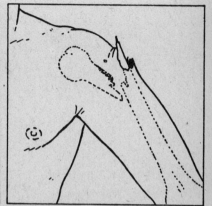

Fig. 3

wound leading down to the fracture, or the bone itself may protrude through the skin (Fig. 3). This will allow blood to escape,
and germs to enter the wound.

With both closed and open fractures, there may be varying
degrees of damage to surrounding tissue or nearby organs.

Treatment—general

A From the clues available, decide that there is (or may be) a
broken bone.

B Cover any wound with a sterile dressing held firmly in place;
take care not to move the injury and cause further damage.

C Immobilize the part immediately, by tying it so that further
unnecessary waggling cannot take place.

D Splints can be used for this purpose, but remember the body
itself makes a good splint; a broken arm may be tied to the
body, or a broken leg may be tied to the good leg.

E When a fracture is suspected, nothing whatsoever should be
given by mouth. (The casualty may need an anaesthetic,
which cannot be given for four hours after eating or drinking.)

Treatments for special parts

SKULL

Fracture of the skull (the top of the head, or brain box) is often
associated with brain damage, and is therefore dealt with in the
chapter on unconsciousness (page 59).

FACE

The bones of the face, and in particular, the lower jaw, are quite
vulnerable.

77

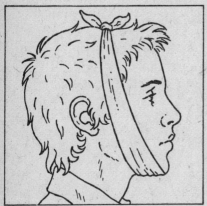

Fig. 4

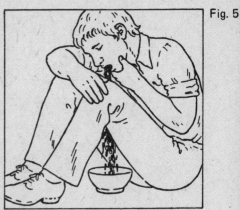

Fig. 5

Treatment

A The bones of the face are best left to a specialist, and apart from covering wounds and stopping bleeding no other action is desirable.

B A broken jaw will waggle unless supported and this is dangerous. Support the jaw with a bandage looped carefully under the jaw and over the top of the head (Fig. 4).

C Face and jaw injuries may be complicated by blood and fluid falling to the back of the throat, so the head should be tilted forward, preferably over a bowl (Fig. 5).

D Keep the breathing passage clear.

E If the casualty is unconscious turn him into the Recovery Position (see page 34).

F Send for an ambulance.

BACKBONE OR SPINE

A broken back is extremely serious because the spinal cord (the main nerve to the lower parts of the body and the legs) is contained in a canal running right through the backbone. If this cord is damaged, severe paralysis may result. If conscious, the casualty may experience severe pain in the back, and there may be numbness, with loss of control of the body downwards from the injured spot.

Treatment

A Ask, 'Can you move your ankles and toes?' (or 'wrists and fingers' if you think the damage is high in neck region).

B Test the limbs by touching them and watching for loss of feeling. If there is no movement or feeling you must assume there is some damage to the spinal cord. If there is movement and feeling but you still suspect a broken spine, play safe and treat for a broken spine.

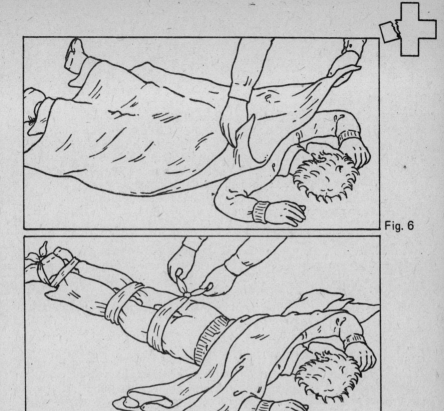

Fig. 6

Fig. 7

C Warn casualty to lie still.
D Do not move away from casualty.
E Call for a doctor or skilled help.
F Cover casualty with coat or blanket (Fig. 6).
If doctor or other help is too far away, proceed (additionally) as follows:
G Place a pad between casualty's ankles and bandage the feet together figure-of-eight-wise.
H Place more pads between knees and thighs and tie the legs together at the knees and thighs, using broad fold bandages (Fig. 7).
I Arrange for removal to hospital.

CHEST

The chest is a cage protecting the heart and lungs. A broken rib does not usually show many outward signs of a fracture, but there is a sharp pain in the chest which becomes worse when breathing deeply or rolling over in bed. If the broken rib should pierce a lung, blood—bright red and frothing—may be coughed up. A penetrating wound, such as a stab wound, could also produce bleeding from the mouth. An open wound in the chest wall will suck air in as the lungs move: this is very dangerous.

79

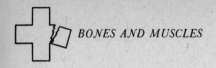

Treatment

A If a broken rib is suspected gently support the arm on the injured side in a sling. See Chapter 2, Fig. 6, page 25.
B If there is a 'sucking' wound (this could be caused by an open fracture), cover the wound immediately to keep the air out; a piece of polythene or a polythene bag, held firmly in position with adhesive tape or a triangular bandage, is ideal.
C Lay the casualty down and incline towards the injured side.
D Arrange for urgent transfer to hospital.

UPPER LIMBS

The arm is anchored across the chest by the collar bone in the front and by the shoulder blade at the back. The shoulder blade is rarely broken.

Treatment

A If a fracture of the shoulder blade is suspected, support the arm on the injured side in a sling.
B Arrange for transfer to hospital.

COLLAR BONE

This is much more prone to injury. The casualty will complain of pain and will often hold the arm at the elbow and incline his head to the injured side, as this gives relief. There may also be swelling over the collar bone.

Treatment

A Support arm in a sling.
B Arrange for transfer to hospital.

FOREARM AND UPPER ARM, WRIST AND HAND

Here the clues are pain and swelling, and in the case of fracture the arm may look misshapen and may also be waggling.

Treatment

A Cover any wounds arising from open fractures first.
B If the elbow will bend, place the arm across the chest with plenty of padding between the chest and the injured part.
C Place the arm in a sling.
D Give extra support by placing a broad bandage over the sling and around the body (Fig. 8).
E If the elbow will not bend, or the elbow joint is affected, bandage the arm to the body in the most comfortable position, over padding.
F Arrange for transfer of casualty to hospital.

HIPS AND PELVIS

80 The pelvis is a platform at the lower end of the trunk, with the

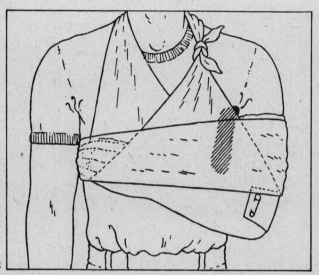

Fig. 8

spine going upwards and the legs downwards, from it. It also en-
circles the bladder which may be damaged if these bones are
broken. The clues are pain, a desire to pass water and inability to
stand up.

Treatment

A Lay casualty down comfortably.
B Warn him *not* to pass water.
C Arrange for removal to hospital—on a stretcher.
D If the journey is long or over rough ground the legs may be tied
together (with separating pads) at the knees and ankles (Fig. 7).
A wide bandage should be placed around the hips for extra
comfort.

LOWER LIMBS

The leg bones are commonly broken, and as they are large bones,
particularly the thigh bones, fractures are often accompanied by
considerable shock. The clues to look for are pain, swelling, misshapen limb, inability to move or stand, and the shock symptoms
of pale face and fast but weak pulse.

Treatment

A First cover any wounds arising from open fractures.
B If the bones are protruding, on no account attempt to push
them back in.
C Support the injured leg and gently move the good leg towards
it, placing padding between them.

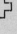

81

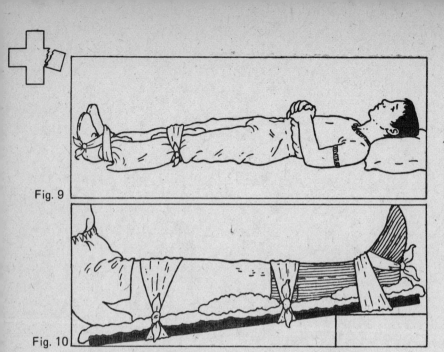

Fig. 9

Fig. 10

D Tie the legs together at the ankles and knees (Fig. 9).
E If the kneecap is broken or a fracture suspected, sit the casualty up, supporting his back.
F Prepare a well-padded splint (if possible long enough to extend from the buttocks to below the heel), and tie at the ankle, just below the knee, and at the thigh (Fig. 10).
G Arrange for transfer to hospital.

Dislocations

We have talked about moveable joints which give a rotating or hinging action. When a bone breaks close to one of these moveable joints it can be complicated by a dislocation. This happens when the two bones meeting at the joint become unattached (and, of course, dislocation can occur whether a bone breaks or not). The clues are:
1 The casualty suffers sickening pain.
2 The joint is misshapen and swollen.
3 The joint is fixed.
Broken and dislocated bones need to be immobilized as soon as possible to stop broken ends from doing more damage, and to reduce pain and shock.

Treatment

A If in any doubt that a bone is fractured, treat as a fracture. Don't take any risks.
B On no account attempt to put the bones back in place.
C Support and bandage the injury securely in the most comfortable position.
D Comfort casualty and get him to a doctor or hospital.

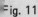

Fig. 11

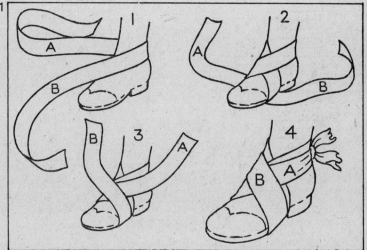

Sprains

These happen when a joint is wrenched and the ligaments around it are torn. The clues are:
1 Pain in the joint, especially when moving.
2 The joint is swollen.
3 Bruising will develop later.

Treatment

A Make casualty comfortable.
B Uncover the joint, pad well and bandage firmly.
C However, if an ankle is sprained, a tight-fitting shoe should be kept on and the bandage applied over it (Fig. 11).
D Comfort casualty and make him rest until he can be removed to hospital or doctor.

Strains

A strain is a stretched or pulled muscle, and the clues are:
1 A sharp pain coming on suddenly.
2 Swelling of injured part.
3 Onset of cramp—sometimes severe.

Treatment

A Make casualty comfortable.
B Support the injured part.
C Comfort casualty and make him rest until he can be removed to hospital or doctor.

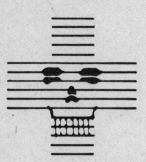

Chapter 9

Poisons

Poisons are substances or gases which when taken into the body in sufficient quantity will harm or destroy life. They can enter the body in three ways:

1 Through the lungs.
2 Through the skin.
3 By mouth.

Poisoning through the lungs is dealt with under Breathing (see pages 45–6). Here then, we deal only with poisons that enter the body through the skin or by the mouth, whether accidentally or intentionally. Poisons which arise from contact come from certain horticultural and agricultural pesticides, and treatment for these conditions has been included. Most poisoning is accidental, and it is vital to take sensible precautions against accidents.

Some important don'ts

Although mentioned already in Chapter 1, a few of these precautions are repeated here for the sake of emphasis. We start with this list because it also includes things which are sometimes attempted as treatments but which should not be used as they are highly dangerous.

1　Never leave tablets or medicines within reach of children (Fig. 1). Keep them in a locked cabinet, or well out of reach (eg on top of a wardrobe).

2　Never store tablets or medicines for long periods. They deteriorate and any surplus at the end of a course of treatment should be returned to the supplier (chemist or doctor) or flushed down the lavatory.

3　Never take drugs in the dark—*always* read the label before taking or giving medicine.

4　Never pour harmful liquids into lemonade or other drink bottles. Children will recognize the bottle and drink the contents.

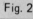

5   Never keep domestic cleaners and detergents under the sink where toddlers can find them (Fig. 2). (By the way, bleach and lavatory cleaners when mixed together do not produce a cleaner lavatory, but do produce a toxic gas which if inhaled is poisonous.)
6   Never make a casualty vomit: never give large quantities of salt water.
7   Never give anything by mouth (unless the mouth is burnt and the casualty is conscious).
8   Never attempt to give anything by mouth if casualty is unconscious.
9   Never wait for a casualty who has swallowed a petroleum preparation to vomit: casualty should be put in the Recovery Position (see page 34) *from the beginning*, with head lower than heart.
10 Never give or take any tablets, especially sleeping tablets, with alcohol—the combination may be fatal.

Fig. 1

Fig. 2

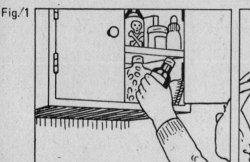

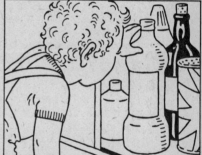

Common poisons

A few of the more common poisons encountered in everyday life are illustrated in Fig. 3. They are:
1 Berries and seeds.
2 Fungi: toadstools.
3 Decomposing food.
4 Strong chemicals: paraffin, petrol, bleaches, weedkillers, chemical fertilizers.
5 Medicines: aspirin, sleeping tablets, tranquillizers, iron tablets.
6 Animal bait: rat and mouse poisons.
7 Alcohol.
8 Green potatoes. (It is not generally appreciated how dangerous green potatoes can be. They can cause colic, vomiting and eventually diarrhoea, possibly followed by collapse.)

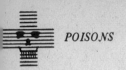

Fig. 3

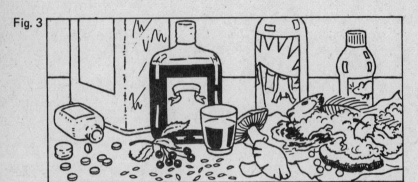

General Treatment

The casualty may be conscious or unconscious, and if the former, may be able to help somewhat with your task.

A While casualty is conscious try to discover what has been swallowed, how much, and when.

B If there are any tablets, empty bottles or cartons near the casualty, keep them for examination in hospital. This may help to identify the poison swallowed.

C Examine the casualty's mouth. If there is evidence of burning and the casualty can swallow, give him as much milk or water as he can drink.

D Should the casualty vomit—catch the vomit in a dish or polythene bag and keep for examination in hospital. Again it may help in identifying the poison swallowed.

E Get the casualty to hospital as quickly as possible.

If the casualty is unconscious or becomes unconscious while in your care:

A First check breathing. If it has stopped, immediately start the Kiss of Life. But if casualty's mouth and lips are burnt, *do not* use the Kiss of Life method; here artificial respiration must be administered (see pages 44–5).

B If casualty is still breathing, place him in the Recovery Position (see page 34) with his lower limbs raised. (A child could be placed over your knee in a slight 'head down' position, during transfer to hospital.)

C Continue to watch casualty's breathing. Many poisons will stop the casualty from breathing.

D Take the casualty to hospital as quickly as possible.

Poisoning through the skin

Today many pesticides, especially those used by nurserymen and farmers, may contain potent chemicals (eg malathion) which, if they come in contact with the skin, are capable of being taken into the body, with disastrous results.

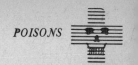
Clues

1 Known contact or contamination with a pesticide.
2 Development of shivering, twitching and fits.
3 Casualty gradually becomes unconscious.

Treatment

A Wash the contaminated area thoroughly with cold water.
B Carefully remove any contaminated clothing, taking care not to touch the chemical yourself.
C Reassure the casualty, lie him down and encourage him to stay still and quiet.
D Arrange for transfer to hospital as soon as possible.
E Keep the casualty cool; apply a cold pad to the forehead and sponge back of neck, spine and body with cold water.
F Encourage casualty to drink as much cool fluid as possible.
G Watch for twitching and fits developing.
H If casualty becomes unconscious, check breathing and place casualty in the Recovery Position (see page 34).
I Always keep the poison container. It may have notes for treatment, but it is also important for your doctor to see it.

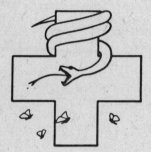

Chapter 10

Bites and stings

Bites and stings should always be taken seriously as their effect may vary from one person to another and there is often a danger of consequential poisoning or disease as distinct from the immediate discomfort: for example, tetanus may ensue from a simple garden or farmyard cut or from the prick of a thorn; mosquito bites can lead to malaria; rabies can follow the bite of a dog, cat or one of a number of wild animals; severe jellyfish stings can cause death. Here are some of the more common occurrences of bites and stings, and the treatment—which is quite simple—for comforting and caring for the casualty.

Dog and cat bites

In countries affected by rabies, all bites must be reported and proper treatment sought either from a doctor or special clinic. Usually bites from pets are unintentional and not very severe, but serious bites can occur when separating fighting animals. In the country, bites from smaller wild animals do occur from time to time. Their treatment is the same as for bites from domestic animals, but they can become septic rapidly.

Treatment
A Wash the wound with soap in clean, running water.
B Dab dry and apply a dry sterile dressing.
C If bleeding is severe, this must be stopped by direct pressure of thumb or finger until a firm sterile dressing can be applied that will control the loss of blood.
D The casualty must be taken or sent to hospital.
E If the wound is gaping after washing, a sterile dressing should be applied and the casualty hurried to hospital for treatment.
F In all cases of bites, a check on the casualty's anti-tetanus injection is necessary.

Scratches, especially from cats

The treatment is generally as for bites. However, there are occasions, fortunately rare, when a cat scratches an eye. This can be extremely painful and cause permanent loss of sight.

Treatment

A Close the eyelids and place a small sterile dressing over the eye to keep it shut.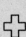

B Take or send the casualty to hospital preferably an eye hospital as soon as possible.

Snake bites

Most snakes only bite if provoked and symptoms in the case of venomous snakes may take some time to develop. The bites of different species require different treatments, thus it is important to identify the snake so that the appropriate antivenene can be given. If the snake is identified as being deadly it is essential to get the casualty to hospital or a treatment centre at the earliest possible moment. If you are uncertain about the identification of the snake, say so at the treatment centre. Don't guess. In such cases, it is safer to give a general antivenene than the wrong one. Most snake bites occur on the limbs.

Treatment

A Lay the casualty down and speak reassuringly to him. Usually the casualty is very frightened and upset by the bite, even though his life may not be in danger.

B Wash the wound well with soap and water, clearing away any venom that remains on the skin near the wound.

C Cover the wound with a sterile dressing.

D Immobilize injured part using a constrictive bandage, which should be loosened every 20 minutes for 30 seconds. Keep the limb in a hanging position.

E Arrange for instant and urgent transfer to hospital (with the dead snake if possible).

F Should the casualty become unconscious, turn him into the Recovery Position (see page 34), and maintain a clear airway.

G Should the casualty show signs of failing breath, or should the breathing stop, then the Kiss of Life or artificial respiration must immediately be started (see pages 43–4 and 44–5). If the heart stops, then heart massage must immediately be started in conjunction with the Kiss of Life (see pages 46–9).

H It should be noted that all hospitals throughout the world which have an Accident and Emergency Department normally keep a stock of anti-venom serum for bites from indigenous poisonous snakes.

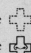

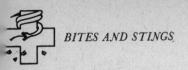

Insects and plants

As with snakes, it is important to identify the cause of the bite or sting and establish if the casualty is aware of any allergy.

Treatment

A When possible, remove the sting from the skin.
B Wash with clean cold water.
C If blistering occurs, prick with a needle (sterilized in a flame or by immersion in boiling water).
D When the fluid has run out of the blister cover the area with a firm dry dressing.

Complications can occur if the sting from a wasp or bee is sustained in the mouth or on the tongue. Swelling will occur and can block the airway, causing difficulty in breathing.

Treatment

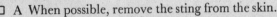

A Give the casualty ice cubes to suck.
B Call for a doctor or for an ambulance to get casualty to hospital.
C Should the casualty become unconscious soon after being stung, place him in the Recovery Position (see page 34).
D Clear the airway.
E If casualty is already unconscious when discovered, carry out stages C and D before B.

TICKS

These small blood-sucking parasites can be destroyed by repeated dressing of affected parts with methylated spirit.

SPIDERS

A number of dangerous species of spider exist in different countries throughout the world and deaths have been recorded. Some antivenenes are available.

Signs

1 Severe swelling around bite.
2 Localized pain.
3 Profuse sweating, shivering and weakness.
4 Casualty may become semi-conscious for several days.
5 The bite itself may become ulcerated.

Treatment

A Apply a constrictive bandage between the bite and the body, using a firm bandage, or if none available, a belt or braces. Wind firmly around the limb in one place.
B Squeeze the bite to force out the poison.

C Loosen the constrictive bandage every 20 minutes for 30 seconds.
D Make casualty rest.
E If possible collect spider in a jar.
F Seek medical advice.

Dangerous marine creatures

SHARK

Severe injuries usually result from encounters with sharks, and safety precautions are essential in shark-infested waters. Treatment appears on page 52.

JELLYFISH

The body's response to jellyfish sting can vary from minor local reaction to large weals, severe pain and even death, which may occur quite swiftly.

Treatment

A Apply calamine cream or lotion, or a paste made of bicarbonate of soda and cold water.
B For severe reactions, seek medical aid urgently.

PORTUGUESE MAN OF WAR

The severity of pain depends upon the amount of poison injected and the state of health of the casualty.

Signs

These vary from slight stinging to cramp, nausea and difficulty in breathing.

Treatment

A Swab the area liberally with alcohol (methylated spirit, brandy or whisky) to which a little vinegar has been added to acidify.
B Do not rub, or apply sand or fresh water.
C Once stinging is inactive, remove any gelatinous strands from the flesh with cloth or soft paper.
D In severe cases seek medical aid.

OCTOPUS

Even the smallest octopus, which may readily be found in a shallow rock pool, can give a fatal bite. *Never* handle an octopus. A bite will readily produce paralysis, respiratory failure and death. There is as yet no antivenene.

SEA URCHINS

There are several types of sea urchin to be found, and in some

91

parts of the world they are considered a great delicacy. Their spines can break off into the skin tissues, causing a burning sensation and intense numbness in the area. The wounds are slow to heal and there is a high risk of infection. Gloves should therefore be worn when handling them.

Treatment

A Remove spines as soon as possible.
B Cover wound with a dry dressing.
C Seek medical advice.

CORAL CUTS

Coral is razor sharp and may cause large deep cuts which readily become infected, are slow to heal and tend to form ulcers.

Treatment

A Clean promptly with methylated spirit.
B Remove all foreign debris.
C Cover with a dressing.
D Seek medical advice.

CONE-SHAPED SHELLS

A snail-like creature housed in an attractive cone-shaped shell is to be found on some beaches of the southern hemisphere. This creature is capable of injecting a very potent poison through a minute hollow-barbed harpoon inside the shell. *Never* handle these shells, as the bite can be fatal and there is no known antidote.

Treatment

A Watch casualty's breathing carefully and carry out Kiss of Life and heart massage as necessary (see pages 43–4 and 46–9).
B Seek medical aid urgently.

Chapter II

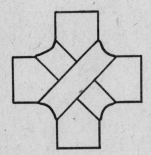

Superficial wounds

Cuts and grazes seem to happen all the time—a common cause in the kitchen is opening tinned food, and for children, simply falling over during impetuous actions—usually playing games. Here we are talking about cuts and grazes that need attention but which do not seem serious enough to take to the doctor. But there is one exception. A very small wound can be very deep, as for example, when the casualty has stepped on a nail, and then he must be seen by a doctor with a view to anti-tetanus treatment. Quite often debris, dirt and infection are carried down into the depth of such a wound and can cause problems. The aim of the treatment is to promote healing and prevent the entry of infection into the wound.

Two don'ts to remember

Wounds heal naturally, and certainly for the less serious ones it is a good rule not to apply ointments, creams or lotions but to let nature do its own work. Also, *do not* touch the part of a dressing that will be applied to the wound; handle dressings lightly by the corners only.

Dressing minor wounds

A Reassure and comfort the casualty, giving extra attention if the casualty is a child.

B Sit the casualty down, preferably in the kitchen, where there is almost always a clean working surface, a supply of hot water, and a washable floor.

C Without touching it, examine the wound.

D Collect first aid box.

E If wound is still bleeding and nothing (like glass) is stuck in it, immediately apply a dressing and press firmly over the wound for a few minutes.

F If you suspect there may be dirt in the wound, clean a surface

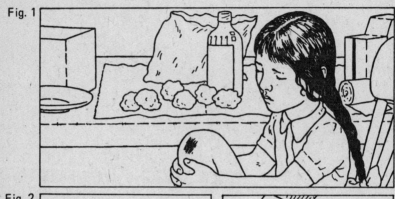

Fig. 1

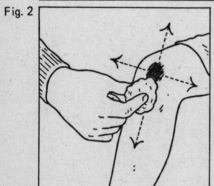

Fig. 2

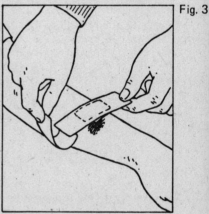

Fig. 3

on which to work and then wash your hands and dry them thoroughly, using clean towel or paper towels. Cover the working top with a clean piece of kitchen paper.

G Open first aid box and lay out required equipment as follows: a number of cotton wool swabs; if antiseptic lotion is to be used, *dilute it* according to manufacturer's instructions (soap and water is, however, just as effective); final dressing, with either adhesive tape or bandage to secure; a paper bag or newspaper for used dressings. These preparations are illustrated in Fig. 1.

H Should the wound and surrounding area be very dirty, it is best to wash the area thoroughly under a gently running tap, using soap as necessary. Clean the outer area surrounding the wound first, then finally the wound itself. If the wound needs further cleaning, use the cotton wool swabs, working from the centre of the wound outwards, and using each swab once only (Fig. 2). Each swab should be damp, not dripping wet and should be discarded into paper bag or newspaper after use.

I After cleaning, dry the wound in the same fashion—the drying of wounds is most important, because if left wet they rapidly become unhealthy and are prone to infection.

J Remember wounds heal best naturally and do not need smothering in ointments and lotions. Small cuts do well simply covered by a suitably-sized adhesive dressing. Take care not to touch the part of the dressing that will cover the wound. When applying the dressing to a cut secure one side first (Fig. 3) and apply a little pressure as you draw the dressing over the cut to secure the other side. This will bring the cut surfaces together and produce a less noticeable scar when healing takes place.

K For larger wounds larger dressings are required. The wound should be covered with a square of sterile gauze, taking care to handle by the corners only. The gauze should be secured with adhesive tape or bandage.

L Burn used dressings, wash hands and put away first aid equipment.

M Remember to replenish first aid box as necessary.

Renewal of dressings

This is not necessary until the original dressing becomes soiled, wet or loose.

A Collect first aid equipment and prepare dressing materials *as before* according to dressing for minor wounds.

B Remove soiled dressing and place directly into paper bag.

C Wash your hands and carry out dressing as before.

D If there is no discharge from the wound do not clean it—just cover it with the new dressing as in dressing for minor wounds.

E If you are at all concerned about the wound you should seek a doctor's advice.

F Wash hands and put away first aid equipment.

The routine for dealing with minor cuts and grazes may be summarized as follows:

A Comfort and reassure casualty and sit him down.

B Collect equipment and prepare working surface.

C Wash hands.

D Open equipment and lay out materials.

E Clean and dry wound thoroughly.

F Cover wound with dressing.

G Clear up, wash hands and replace equipment.

H Replenish equipment.

Section III

Special Circumstances

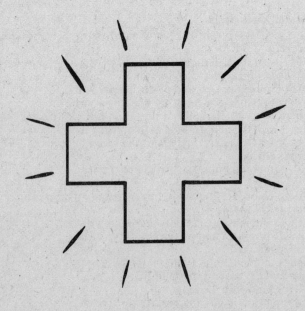

Chapter 12

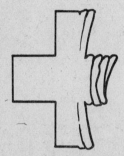

Road accidents

The injuries sustained in road accidents must fall into one or other of the categories already described in earlier chapters—there will be wounds, bleeding, fractures, burns, shock and very often unconscious casualties. But two things will be very different: firstly, the situations in which road accidents occur; and secondly, the severity of injuries due to the force of impact. There is also the tendency for road accidents—especially those occurring on motorways at high speeds—to involve several casualties and for those casualties to suffer multiple injuries.

The road accident and you

There is the possibility that either you personally are involved in an accident, or you are one of the first to come on the scene of an accident. Should you be involved in an accident and be injured, there is nothing, or very little indeed, that you can do to help; someone else must take over. A wise precaution for *every* motorist is to have essential directory details on a card kept in the dashboard pocket—simply a note of your name, address and telephone number.

It may be, however, that you are not injured personally, and you may want to start organizing the situation. But remember that you will inevitably suffer shock, and this may impair your judgement. Also you may not be the best judge of priorities. If your wife, husband, son or daughter has a broken arm it may be natural to alleviate the pain with a sling while an unconscious casualty with a blocked airway is dying for lack of breath. So the rule is to offer help, but *not* to take charge unless there is no alternative.

Arriving on the scene

When a road accident happens, there are instantly a number of possible hazards. The accident may block the road completely or

97

partially, and debris or casualties may be scattered in the path of oncoming traffic. This confused situation may be worsened by having morbid spectators either stopping and causing congestion or driving slowly by, not concentrating on their driving. The first thing you must ask yourself is 'Can I be of help if I stop?' This decision must be made in a matter of moments, and here are the considerations to help you.

1 If ambulance or police are already on the scene, do not stop or stare, but drive on.
2 Has the situation obviously been taken over by other motorists, ie flagging down fast vehicles and directing traffic past the situation? If so, you can assume they will also have sent for help, and unless you have a first aid box (or a flashing lamp or torch for use by night) in the car, you should drive on.
3 Does the accident still need an organizer?
4 Have I a first aid box in my car?

Deciding to stop at an accident

If you decide to stop, remember these priorities.
1 Concentrate on your driving, not the accident, until you stop.
2 Watch your mirror for other motorists—don't brake hard when someone is coming up fast behind you and possibly not concentrating.
3 Pull *ahead* of the accident and park *off* the road if possible. You may be tempted to park your car behind the accident as a shield. Although this might be an advantage in the city, it is highly dangerous on a motorway, so pull ahead, park and walk back. *Always* park on the near-side of the road.
4 Remember to take your first aid box (and lamp or torch by night) with you.

Organizing the situation

Once on the scene, there are further priorities to consider. To save further damage being done, it is essential that they are tackled in the right order.
1 Warn oncoming traffic. Ideally warning triangles should be set up at 300, 200 and 100 metres from the accident, but it is unlikely that these signs will be available until the police arrive, in which case get helpers to stand at these points to flag down oncoming traffic. Tell them to stand at the side of the road, not in it. The warning at 300 metres is the most important.
For stopping distances, you should refer to the figures issued by motoring organizations. Remember that it is very important to give warning at appropriate intervals, as a fast-moving motorist may pass the first and even the second signal before appreciating their significance.

2 Very rapidly size up the situation. Your first task is to get some-one to telephone 999 for emergency services, but before that can be done it is necessary to be able to give essential informa-tion about the accident. Whoever is going to telephone must be able to say
- (A) Where the accident has happened—describe the location as accurately as possible, eg 'On M6 northbound carriage-way about 3 miles north of Exit 14'.
- (B) The number of vehicles involved (if more than three say 'multiple').
- (C) Type of vehicles involved if unusual, eg petrol tanker, chemical carrier, bus.
- (D) Number of injured (if more than 4, approximate, eg 'about half-a-dozen,' 'about a dozen', or 'a bus-load' – don't stop to count.
- (E) Details of any casualties trapped.
- (F) If there is a fire or special danger of fire.
- (G) Any other relevant information.
- (H) The exchange (or code) and number of the telephone being used.

3 When phoning 999, helper should ask for all the emergency services required at the same time, eg, as appropriate, ambu-lance, police, fire brigade, and fire (rescue) service, and say which is most urgent.

4 If you have a helper available for the purpose, and it is necessary, post this helper on traffic control duty.

5 Take safety precautions:
- (A) Switch off engines (and, if there is time, disconnect batteries) of vehicles involved in the accident.
- (B) Apply handbrakes of involved vehicles, or place chocks under wheels.
- (C) Extinguish fire if one has started, using fire extinguishers, blankets or soil. But be careful of exploding petrol tanks. (Remember that vehicles can be crushed in multiple accidents, and petrol may pour onto the road or leak slowly as a result. Either may lead to a sudden explosion.)
- (D) Do not smoke, and stop others from doing so.
- (E) Make sure that you personally and other helpers are not in danger (eg from oncoming traffic). No extra casualties are needed!

6 *Do not drag casualties clear of vehicles* unless there is immediate danger (eg fire, or vehicle finely balanced and liable to topple onto casualty).

7 *Leave the movement of severely injured casualties until arrival of emergency services*, but on motorways, a casualty who has been thrown clear of a vehicle must be moved immediately from the traffic lanes onto the hard shoulder. This involves considerable danger to both helper and casualty. Casualty must be handled

as carefully as possible, because he must be moved before diagnosis is possible.

Dealing with the casualties

Having quickly organized the situation so that no further damage will be done and help is on its way, you can turn your attention to the casualties. The Help Routine is now your guide, but you may have the additional problem of distinguishing between the injuries to a number of casualties, in which case you have to decide on the priorities for treatment. This is your drill:

A However serious the situation may be, don't panic—keep calm and cool. Examine unconscious casualties first, starting with the Shake, Shout and Pinch routine (see page 31) and continuing from the head downwards.

B Apply the See, Hear and Feel routine (see pages 31–2). This means firstly *looking* to size up the situation, and then to identify visual clues to the condition of the casualties; secondly, *asking* witnesses and conscious casualties to say what has happened and to describe their injuries or condition; and thirdly, *feeling* for swellings, bumps and lumps which will indicate injuries under the skin.

C Summarize all the clues and make your diagnosis.

D In casualties where breathing has stopped, apply the Kiss of Life immediately (see pages 43–4). Also check heart-beat (pulse) and if there is none, remove casualty from car onto ground and start heart massage immediately (see pages 46–9).

E For applying Kiss of Life and heart massage simultaneously, see page 48.

F After breathing and heart-beat, turn your attention to bleeding and take steps to stop it (see pages 50–2).

G Immobilize bone damage to prevent further movement. If casualty complains of neck injury, fold a newspaper and place around the neck, and secure with a bandage or scarf (Fig. 1). Remember not to tie too tightly!

Fig. 1

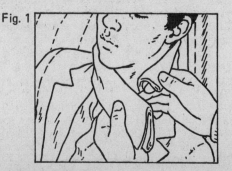

H Encourage and comfort casualties where possible, keeping them warm with rugs or spare clothing. Give no alcohol ever. Give no food or liquid to unconscious casualties or casualties who are likely to need an anaesthetic.

I Look for the effects of shock and concussion among casualties and apparently unharmed passengers in collision vehicles, and look around for any who may have wandered off and collapsed. For early treatment for shock, see page 40.

J When medical help arrives, report concisely on the situation and the individual casualties. The information that you can pass on at this stage may save a life.

K Before leaving the scene of an accident it is wise to confirm that control has been effectively passed over by you to the authorities.

L Remember to collect up all your own equipment and take it back to your car.

M Don't spoil it all by pulling up at the next pub for a large brandy and then being asked to do a breath test.

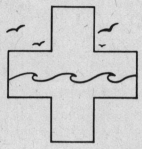

Chapter 13

Holiday and sports injuries

Fitness of mind and body depends on leisure and healthy exercise; practically everyone maintains his or her fitness by taking holidays, and many also participate in some kind of sporting activity. Obviously injuries may be sustained during holidays and games, and they must affect the body in the same ways as those already described. But once again the circumstances in which they happen are going to be different. When a thousand miles from home in a foreign country, you cannot dial 999; when you are in a yacht 50 miles out at sea, you cannot nip into a chemist's shop for surgical supplies; and you may be beyond help of any kind lying injured in a mountain pass if elementary precautions have not been taken to alert authorities or friends to your whereabouts and intentions.

So holidays have a number of attendant risks. Even lazing in the sun in some foreign clime has its hazards: serious sunburn can be sustained long before the casualty actually starts to feel discomfort, and he may also suffer sunstroke to boot. The rule is to relax and have your fun without over-indulging in unaccustomed exercise, sunbathing, or unusual food.

And then there are holidays where the central theme is a sport. On the general field of sports, the participants divide sharply into two groups. Firstly there are those who earn their living playing as professionals, together with those experts, many of them amateurs, who play representative sports for their club, league, county or country. Secondly there are those who play games for exercise or simply for fun.

The first of these groups, the professionals and experts, have the advantage that behind them there is a carefully organized back-up consisting of training programme, gymnasium, trainers, doctors and first aid. Also these devoted sportsmen are disciplined to obey a few simple but essential rules. They:

1 train regularly and maintain a condition of complete fitness for their particular sport.

2 know, understand and obey implicitly the rules of their game.

3 use only equipment and clothing which is suitable and in excellent condition.
4 use their common sense.
5 never take risks, either with themselves or others.

The second group, the amateurs or non-experts, who play for exercise and fun, often disobey these rules, although there are of course exceptions. There would be far fewer sports accidents if only the enthusiastic amateurs would follow the example of the professionals. Instead, they tend to throw themselves into sudden activity, resulting in overuse of muscles and tendons. They forget that in some sports the players are pushing their bodies to the limits of their endurance and that unless the body is toned up to meet the strain, something is bound to crack. They fail to realize that they may be wearing very little lightweight clothing which may make examination easier but provides less to keep them warm. Certainly they overlook the fact that their pulse, or heartbeat, and breathing rates will increase considerably, bringing nearer the point of exhaustion beyond which damage and suffering will follow. The primary rule is *use your common sense and don't do too much.*

Logic will tell you the type of injuries normally associated with different types of sport, and such injuries will usually be caused by:
1 Overuse, leading to pulled muscles, strains and sprains, and cramps.
2 Body contact, as in football, rugby and boxing.
3 Conveyance, as in riding, skiing, motoring.
4 Apparatus, as with cricket balls, hockey sticks, trampolines.
5 Natural hazards, as in climbing, pot-holing and water sports.

Here is a short review of sports in their main groups, with some of their hazards.

Soccer and rugby

These two very popular sports account for over 40% of all sports injuries. Knees, ankles and legs are particularly vulnerable in both sports. Knees are always being damaged and one in every four sports injuries involves the knee. Rugby football has additional hazards for the back, arms and ribs. The injuries arise almost entirely from body contact in fast-moving collisions, tackling, tripping and falling. Very occasionally serious damage is done in collision with goal posts. The range of injuries from all these causes includes broken bones, dislocations, sprains and bruises, wounds with bleeding, and occasionally unconsciousness, in addition to those arising from overuse of the body.

Racket, bat and stick games

Cricket, tennis, squash, hockey, and golf all come under this

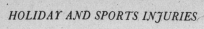

heading, and the injuries fall into three groups:

1 Injuries caused by the racket, bat, stick or club.
2 Injuries caused by missiles.
3 Overuse of the body.

Perhaps hockey and ice-hockey sticks are the worst offenders, and are frequently responsible for wounds, broken bones, winding and unconsciousness. Hard balls, such as cricket and golf balls, cause similar injuries. The so-called tennis elbow is a good example of damage arising through overuse: joints, muscles, ligaments and tendons are all vulnerable. Perhaps shooting should be included in this grouping because of the missile—a cartridge-load of small shot. Where accidents happen the shot usually penetrates the flesh without much bleeding, but surgical shock will ensue. After dealing with the priorities the casualty should be removed to hospital immediately.

Athletics

Athletics and gymnastics are more competitive and individual than games with opposing teams or participants. Usually the athlete is a solo performer or has his lane for running reserved for him. He is nevertheless susceptible to injury from three causes:

1 Accident with apparatus, such as vaulting horses, springboards, and parallel bars.
2 Pole jumping, javelin throwing, shot putting, weight lifting and other sports requiring use of special equipment, and needing exceptional muscular strength.
3 Overuse of the body.

Athletes drive themselves to the limit of their endurance, and the resulting overuse will cause damage to joints, muscles, ligaments and tendons, and to strain on the heart which can lead in turn to collapse and unconsciousness. Broken bones, dislocations, wounds, bleeding and unconsciousness can all follow accidents with apparatus and special equipment.

Wrestling comes into this category and normally the rules of the sport prevent accidents occurring in the course of the sport itself. Exceptionally, combatants may fall badly—sometimes out of the ring—and this can lead to any of the injuries mentioned from using apparatus and equipment.

Water sports

Water is the common factor in swimming, diving, rowing, surfing, yachting, canoeing, water-skiing and fishing. Accidents in or on the water may involve physical injury during the incident, and can also leave the casualty subject to the two great water hazards, drowning and exposure—sometimes in very cold conditions.

Swimming can be very relaxing, but it is a sport where fitness and obeying the rules are both very important. It needs great strength to swim against strong tides and currents. So never get into situations that are—or may be—dangerous. And remember that cramp on the sportsfield may be very painful, but in the water it can lead to death by drowning. Underwater swimming requires good equipment—make sure that air bottles are fully charged and that all the valves are working. Swim in pairs for safety and watch out for underwater hazards, which are listed, with appropriate treatments, in Chapter 10, under the heading 'Dangerous marine creatures'. Always take safety precautions in shark-infested waters. Bathe only on mesh-protected beaches: listen for the shark bell: leave the water when warned to do so: and avoid wearing white which is said to attract sharks. Treatment for shark bites appears on page 52.

Sailing has its own hazards including swinging booms, flaying ropes, rough weather causing violent movement of the boat, and water washing over the deck. Yachting in open water requires a considerable number of skills, and because of weather changes which spring up without warning and the complicated 'rule of the road' in coastal waters, which are now very busy, the un-initiated sailor should not venture out to sea. Here it is sufficient to say: take all precautions possible, including the checking of weather reports, and of equipment including sails, auxiliary engines and all equipment. Always have a first aid box aboard and make sure it is fully equipped *before* setting sail; also you should always carry a two-way radio and distress signals. Remember that in an emergency, *you* are the one that has to communicate your needs to the outside world, and the rule is to be as self-sufficient as possible.

The nature of injuries aboard ship is similar to those on land—broken bones, wounds, bleeding, unconsciousness and burns including rope burns. All these conditions and their treatments have been dealt with in Chapters 5 to 8. Beware of fire and of poisonous gases used for cooking (remember they are mostly heavier than air). It is bad enough to suffer injuries aboard ship, but to this can be added exposure, either to a man overboard, or to the complete crew if a vessel becomes immobilized and is forced to drift.

Sports of conveyance

Cars, cycles and motor cycles, horses, planes, and gliders all come into this category. Speed is the common denominator and gives rise to conditions where impact with other fast-moving or static objects will result in multiple injuries, often having a high fire risk. Common injuries include broken bones, wounds and bleeding, spinal injuries, unconsciousness, damage to internal organs and to the brain, sometimes complicated by serious burns.

Winter sports

Very cold weather is a basic necessity for these sports, which include skiing, skating and tobogganning; skating has also become an indoor round-the-year sport. Skiing is essentially a sport requiring good snow and wide-open sloping spaces. It is fast-moving and attracts all the accidents associated with high speed. Nearly three-quarters of all skiing injuries are to the legs, and involve broken bones, and injuries to joints, muscles, ligaments and tendons. The ankles and knees are most prone to joint injury, and the bones of the lower leg are the most frequently broken. Dislocation of the thumb and of the shoulder are perhaps the most common injuries in the upper parts of the body.

EXPOSURE AND FROSTBITE

Shock and collapse will be aggravated by cold exposed conditions and lead on to hypothermia unless early protection and treatment is afforded. Frostbite is a danger in very cold conditions, especially to fingers, toes, ears and nose. Should these extremities become white and numb, do not attempt to rewarm by rubbing with snow, a towel, or your hands.

Treatment

A Warm the frostbitten parts by placing them next to warm parts of the casualty's body or a helper's body.

B Place fingers under armpits; cover nose with cupped hands; feet and toes can be covered with a blanket or placed against a helper's warm back or even armpits.

C Remove rings from fingers and laces from boots or shoes.

D Smoking should not be allowed, but a *small* amount of alcohol could improve the circulation.

E Seek medical advice if any discoloration of skin is noticed.

F *Do not apply direct heat* such as a hot water bottle or hot compress.

G For snow-blindness, keep the casualty quiet in a darkened room.

Big game hunting

The dangers of safari are numerous and cannot all be listed here. Emergency treatments have been specified in earlier chapters for almost all the injuries that may arise. For wounds inflicted by animals, the treatments will be found in the chapters dealing with bleeding, bites and stings; for fractures, burns and poisons there are also special chapters. The most important advice for the big game hunter is to put himself in the care of professionals, use the correct equipment and obey the rules of the game, whether posted on notice boards or communicated by game wardens. And never play with fire, metaphorically or otherwise!

Climbing and pot-holing

These sports are only for very fit and well-trained participants, and yet enthusiastic beginners often seem to become involved in them. It is essential to obey the rules and use equipment which has been properly serviced and inspected before being used each time. Added to the expected injuries from falls (which include broken bones, wounds and bleeding and unconsciousness—often with multiple injuries) are the dangers of exposure and of becoming trapped in confined spaces. The essential pre-requisite is to advise somebody—family, friend, hotel-keeper or police—where you are going and when you expect to return.

Minor conditions

Whilst most of the problems that may arise have been discussed in previous chapters, here are a few minor conditions that have not been dealt with earlier.

STITCH IN THE SIDE

This usually occurs when exercise has been taken too soon after a meal. The pain, which may develop in either side, can be quite severe.

Treatment
A Casualty should stop running or walking and just rest.
B The pain will gradually disappear.
C No other treatment is necessary.

CRAMP

A vice-like pain that occurs suddenly in a muscle. (The calf or thigh muscles are most commonly affected.)

Treatment
The aim is to stretch the painful muscle.
A In the calf—pull the big toe forward towards the shin. Remember to keep the knee straight.
B In the thigh—keep the leg straight and press the knee backwards.
C The pain will gradually disappear.

WINDING

This is caused by a sudden blow to the upper part of the belly (solar plexus). The casualty doubles up with pain.

Treatment
A Allow the casualty to curl up into the position he finds most comfortable.

107

B Leave him to recover in his own good time.

INJURIES TO JOINTS AND MUSCLES

In injuries such as dislocations, sprains and bruising, discomfort can be eased and swelling reduced by the application of a cold compress. This applies also to the major injuries described in Chapter 8.

Treatment

A Soak a towel, face cloth or piece of material in cold water and apply it to the injury as a compress.
B Change the compress every 10 to 15 minutes.
Alternatively:
A From the freezer, take a packet of frozen peas, wrap in a clean dry towel and apply over the injury.
B This compress will retain its coldness for a considerable time.

Excessive heat

This may affect the body in two ways Heat stroke or Heat exhaustion.

HEAT STROKE

Heat stroke can develop quite rapidly when the body is unable to cool itself by sweating and the temperature of the body rises above normal levels. It is likely to happen to people who are suddenly exposed to high temperatures and who do not take adequate precautions. The sensible precautions are:

1 Acclimatization, ie settling in for a day or two before undertaking vigorous holiday activities in hot humid climates.
2 Wearing light loose airy clothing.
3 Using fans to keep air moving.
4 Drinking plenty of cool fluids — 7–10 pints (4–5½ litres) every 24 hours.
5 Adding extra salt to food at meal times (but only if there is a plentiful supply of water).

Clues

Casualty complains of
1 Headache.
2 Feeling very hot.
3 Pulse feels strong and pounding.
4 Casualty may be confused and delirious.
5 Casualty may become unconscious.

Treatment

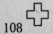

The temperature of the casualty must be reduced quickly:
A Remove clothing.

B Sponge the body using tepid water (cold water will make the casualty shiver and this in turn will produce more heat).
C Apply cold compress to forehead.
D Seek medical advice if temperature does not fall.

HEAT EXHAUSTION

Heat exhaustion may take some time (even a day or two) to develop. It is caused by an excessive loss of salt and water from the body, usually after vigorous exercise on a very hot day but it may also develop in a hot climate or when the body loses a great deal of fluid during an attack of severe diarrhoea and vomiting.

Clues

Casualty complains of
1 Tiredness, headache and possibly cramp in muscles of the limbs and belly (abdomen).
2 The face becomes pale and the skin feels quite cold, clammy and sweaty.
3 Casualty may feel faint and dizzy.
4 The body temperature may remain normal.

Treatment

A Keep the casualty in the shade.
B Give diluted fruit juice to which ½ teaspoon of salt has been added to each pint (½ litre).
C If no improvement, seek medical advice.

Conclusion

In this review of sports and their risks, we have done something to identify the injuries usually sustained in particular games, but little has been said about treatment, and the reason is logical. Organisers of sporting events normally make their own arrangements for first aid, not only for the athletes but also for the spectators, so that the chances of the reader being called upon to help at organised events are usually very remote. It is only in the personal accident situation, such as on holiday or in friendly games and healthy pastimes, that the reader may need to provide first aid, and in Section II of *Help!* we have already told the reader precisely what to do and what not to do.

A good piece of advice if you are British and going abroad is to take with you Certificate ECIII which will entitle you to immediate medical care throughout the Common Market countries under a reciprocal arrangement with the National Health Service in Britain. You can obtain this Certificate by taking your National Insurance number to your local office of the Department of Health and Social Security.

Chapter 14

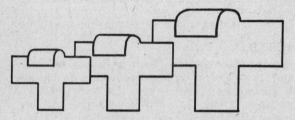

Accidents related to age groups

This chapter has been included to make the reader aware of the different kinds of accidents to which people are prone at different times of their lives—from the cradle to the grave. To some extent, therefore, it supplements Chapter 1, Accidents. It will be seen that most accidents happen to the very young when they are exploring their new world, and to the very old who are frail in mind and body, and have lost the concentration and judgement of their prime. Both these groups need supervision and control. Excessive loss of heat to the body (hypothermia) is dealt with for all age groups at the end of the chapter.

Infants—birth to 5 years

SUFFOCATION

This can take place in a cot or pram and can be prevented by not using pillows in the early years, until the child can turn over on its own. If a baby is found in this condition, instantly send for a doctor, and apply the Kiss of Life and heart massage (for treatment see pages 43–4 and 46–9).

FALLS FROM COT OR PRAM

These can be prevented by securing the infant correctly in an approved harness. When a fall occurs, the infant usually suffers a bump on the head. A wad of lint or gauze soaked in cold water and held over the bump is all that is necessary to control the size of the bump. But if the infant is unconscious, place in the Recovery Position (see page 34) and take him to hospital as soon as possible.

FOREIGN BODIES IN NOSE AND EARS

Toddlers will push all manner of objects into nose and ears: small beads are popular. Only if the foreign body is actually sticking out of the entrance should you attempt to remove it. Using the wrong

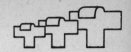

instrument or wrong method may do more damage than leaving it until the child can be treated by a doctor. Foreign bodies can also be swallowed and this causes anxiety, particularly if the nature of the object is not known. If however the object is known to be small and rounded and unlikely to dissolve, no harm will come to the child and the object will emerge from the bowel in due course. But if the object is sharp or jagged, such as a pin, needle or piece of broken glass, take the child to a doctor immediately.

CHOKING

Infants often choke through taking too much food into their mouths or attempting to take a deep breath when eating food. Food then gets stuck in the back of the throat and, if allowed to remain, blocks the airway.

Treatment

A Remove all contents from mouth.
B Turn infant upside down.
C Give a sharp slap across back.
Often A will suffice: use your finger to get to the back of the throat to be sure that all the food is removed from the mouth. At stage B gravity plays a part, and this again may be sufficient to clear the airway. Stage C usually completes the dislodgement of any remaining food.

CUTS

These almost invariably result from the carelessness or stupidity of parents in leaving sharp objects around. (For treatment see page 93–5.)

SCALDS AND BURNS

Again such accidents stem from parental carelessness. The child grabs saucepans on the cooker, or approaches unguarded fires; or just sits surrounded by toys in the hall waiting for mother complete with tray to trip up and pour boiling coffee all over baby. (For treatment see pages 70–2.)

SUNBURN AND SUNSTROKE

Tiny babies should not be left in their prams in direct sunlight. The wearing of synthetic baby clothes or the use of nylon sheets and covers can cause excessive loss of body fluid through sweating. Babies can ill-afford to lose fluid in this way. In very hot weather fluid intake should be increased by giving *small* quantities of water between feeds.

Toddlers should wear light cotton shirts over swimming shorts when playing, especially on the beach. Their skins are so sensitive that they burn very easily; hats should also be worn. Any child

111

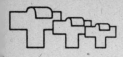

who has been badly burned *must* be seen by a doctor. The early treatment for the very young is the same as for adults (see page 73).

BLOWS ON THE HEAD
Toddlers without exception fall downstairs before they are five and usually hit their heads. Fortunately it is usually just a bump: but in the case of any of the following symptoms, it is advisable to seek medical advice. The child may:
1 Be knocked unconscious—if only for a few seconds.
2 Vomit during the next 24 hours, for no other known reason.
3 Complain of increasing headache.
4 Go to sleep at an unusual time.
5 Complain of being unable to see properly, or have double vision.
6 Have a fit.
Don't wait to 'see what happens'. It may then be too late. Seek medical aid immediately.

FRACTURED COLLAR BONE
 A toddler can fall, pick himself up and go on playing, yet have broken a collar bone. He will become more miserable as the day goes by, and he will not move his arm when being undressed. By now he will be irritable if the arm is moved. The history is always the same: the fall, followed by irritability and a slight swelling and tenderness over the collar bone, and a resistance to movement. The fracture will be confirmed by the doctor or on X-ray at hospital.

NAPPY PINS
These are sometimes driven into babies by hurried or preoccupied mothers. If the skin has simply been pierced, cleaning and covering with a dressing is all that is necessary. If however the pin has passed through the penis or actually gone through the abdominal wall then medical advice must be sought.

POISONING
 Children always suck toys, and paint on wooden and metal toys can cause poisoning, though such cases are rare nowadays. Where suspected it is necessary to take medical advice. (See also Chapter 9, pages 85–6, for swallowing of pills, berries and other possible poisons.)

D AND V (Diarrhoea and Vomiting)
Excessive D and V in a baby or toddler must be taken seriously, as this causes loss of body fluids which cannot be afforded.

Treatment
A Do not give any food.

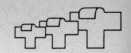

B Give small quantities of water at regular intervals (*not too much* as this will cause the casualty to vomit and make matters worse).

C Seek medical advice.

Children—5 to 10 years

As a child grows older and becomes more adventurous, the injuries become more frequent and more severe. Much the same advice as for toddlers applies to this age group. The foreign bodies inserted into the various orifices of their bodies get bigger and better, and medical advice is essential. The cuts, scalds, blows and broken limbs also tend to be bigger and better. The nose-bleed is a common finding and when occurring frequently, the child should be referred to a doctor.

Young people—10 to 20 years

Injuries to this group tend to be more severe than those to the very young and old. Team games and motor cycles contribute largely to the risks that result in severe head injuries. There is no advice that will stop these accidents happening. Perhaps the consolation is that the power of recovery at this age is very considerable. (See also chapter 13, Holiday and Sports Injuries.)

Adults—20 to 45 years

The injuries and diseases associated with occupations now begin to play a part, and they can, of course, be very varied.

Adults will suffer occupational injuries, sports injuries and car and motor cycle injuries. Women may experience heavy periods, miscarriages and bleeding from childbirth. Treatments for all these conditions are included in the appropriate chapters.

Adults—45 to 65 years

Heart attacks now become more prevalent. (For treatment see pages 64–5.) Also the occasional stroke occurs as the age of 65 is reached. Adults in this age group are prone to all the conditions of the 20–45 year age group, except perhaps for miscarriage and childbirth bleeding.

The elderly aged over 65 years

The problems here are similar to those of the very young. It is largely a matter of being unable to cope. They no longer appreciate danger and attempt foolish projects, such as cleaning windows or putting up curtains, which they are incapable of actually doing, and then they have an accident.

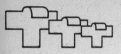

FRACTURE OF HIP BONE (Neck of Femur)

This is a common fracture for the elderly, often caused by tripping over rugs or slipping on polished floors. The symptoms are complaint of pain in the injured hip and inability to move the leg. The casualty will lie with the foot of the injured leg turned outwards, so it is easily diagnosed following a note of the history of the fall. If the casualty is to walk again, an operation is essential and hospitalization is urgently needed. (For treatment see pages 80–1.)

STROKES

The older person has a greater chance of suffering a stroke. (For treatment see pages 62–3.)

FAINTING

 This is common in the elderly and occurs through getting up too quickly from a sitting or lying position, when giddiness is followed by passing out, perhaps only momentarily. However the elderly can fall awkwardly and perhaps knock themselves out. This can be dangerous if it happens, say, after turning on the gas but before lighting it, or when holding a kettle of boiling water. Treatment, when the casualty is discovered, is to place in the Recovery Position (see page 34), and if other injuries are indicated, send casualty to hospital. If it is merely a faint, call a doctor.

SCALDS AND BURNS

These frequently occur simply due to inability to cope with cooking and other kitchen tasks. Also the elderly fail to appreciate the permanent need for fire guards.

NOSE-BLEEDS FROM HIGH BLOOD PRESSURE

High blood pressure is common amongst the very old and consequently they suffer nose-bleeds. This happens suddenly and despite first aid treatment described on pages 53–4, will not stop after a few minutes, but continues and needs plugging by a doctor. Therefore the doctor should be summoned immediately, as only he can do this. Often a large number of towels are necessary to contain the bleeding until the doctor arrives. The casualty becomes distressed at the sight of so much blood, and the blood-stained towels should be kept away from the casualty's vision.

HEART ATTACK

This is a common occurrence in this age group, and is frequently the cause of death, despite the emergency treatment outlined on pages 64–5.

FRACTURED LIMBS

More fractures occur to ankles and wrists in this age group than in

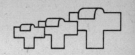

any other. They are due to unsteadiness, leading to falls, especially during the winter when snow and ice are about. (For treatment see pages 80 and 81–2).

ACCIDENTAL POISONING

This arises from taking the wrong tablets and also from forgetting whether they have already taken the prescribed number of tablets or not, and thus taking double doses. Also, due to frailty, an elderly person may drink medicine from the wrong bottle, possibly a poison for use in the garden. (For treatment see pages 85–6.)

ACCIDENTAL COOLING (hypothermia)

This dangerous fall in body temperature occurs particularly in babies, the elderly and the severely handicapped, and also in people who are on drugs or drink excessive amounts of alcohol. Babies are especially susceptible because of their body surface which is large in proportion to their weight. In other cases the condition is usually caused by physical inactivity, or from insufficient clothing or nourishment. Hypothermia can also occur through exposure in a number of outdoor situations, and this is dealt with separately at the end of this chapter.

Clues

In the case of babies, there are three clues to look for:
1 The baby will be unduly quiet.
2 He will refuse food.
3 He will feel deadly cold.
The hands, face and feet may remain a healthy pink, which is misleading.

For other age groups the clues are different, but conform to a pattern:
1 The casualty will be very pale.
2 He will have a slow, weak pulse.
3 He will feel deadly cold.
4 He will be dreamy and slow to react.
5 He will be excessively tired.
6 He will suffer cramp, loss of movement and stumble.
7 He may possibly have fits or become unconscious.
When casualty becomes unconscious, death will almost certainly ensue unless immediate action is taken.

Prevention

The risk of hypothermia may be reduced for babies and adults by:
1 Providing a warm environment.
2 Ensuring that casualty has adequate clothing and food at all times.

115

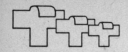

Treatment for babies, the elderly, invalids and special cases

A Prevent further heat loss with blankets and clothes.
B Arrange urgent transfer to hospital.
Do not attempt to give extra heat by using hot-water bottles or electric blankets: this will only cause the blood pressure to drop dangerously.

COLD WET CHILLING

Hikers, pot-holers, mountaineers and other outdoor sportsmen can contract hypothermia from exposure. This comes particularly from cold wet chilling, caused by clothing saturated by mists, rain or perspiration, or by immersion in water.

Prevention

The clues in cold wet chilling are the same as for hypothermia, but prevention can be more objective. For those on land, the following hints may be useful. They should:
1 Dress warmly.
2 Wear additional protective clothing, including hoods (loose waterproofed nylon clothing is excellent—and light).
3 Carry reserve clothing.
4 Have correct supervision and leadership.
5 Let someone know the intended route.
Casualties in cold water (eg after falling overboard) should remember that more deaths are caused through loss of body heat than through drowning. They should always remain still in the water; treading water or swimming around requires energy and will encourage heat loss.

Treatment

A If possible remove wet clothing and dry casualty.
B Wrap casualty in warm blankets.
C Warm casualty by placing in hot bath.
D Encourage heat retention by use of sleeping bags or even large polythene bags. (This is vital if facilities for a hot bath are not available.)

E Arrange urgent transfer to hospital.

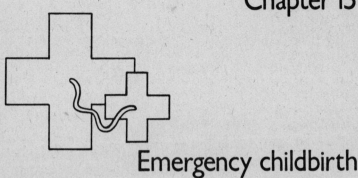

Chapter 15

Emergency childbirth

When you consider that a birth may be—even normally—up to three weeks premature or three weeks overdue, it is perhaps surprising that the vast majority of babies are born in hospital or at home according to plan. But a very considerable number are also born at the most inconvenient times—in trains, aeroplanes, shops and even in the street. The service that even a person with very little knowledge can give to the distressed mother is invaluable. Anyone can be the unwitting witness to this situation, but how much more rewarding to be able to give practical help. There is also the possibility that weather conditions of heavy snow, floods, ice or blizzard or some other crisis will step in to cut off professional help just when it is needed. Life tends to be a little like that! So what could *you* do if faced with an emergency childbirth? The answer is—a lot. By reading the pages of this chapter, you will see how much you can do to give practical assistance to a mother in this situation.

The preliminary routine

The first thing to remember is that childbirth is a perfectly normal event. In its own good time the baby will be born with or without your help. The only unusual circumstance is that it has decided to happen when you are there to help and a doctor or midwife is not. So keep calm and take stock of the situation; if you are anxious or agitated your fears will be apparent to your patient which is bad for her. The preliminary routine to follow is:

A Keep calm (you can panic when it is all a memory!)
B Don't rush around.
C Assess the situation.
D Reassure the patient (and also the husband or other relatives who may be there).
E Contact a doctor or midwife, and if unavailable dial 999 and ask for the flying squad.

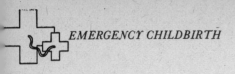
Assessment of the situation

Your first question to the mother must be 'Is this your first baby?' First babies take longer to be born, and in such cases you usually have time on your side. Second and subsequent babies may be born much more quickly, but there is a compensating bonus, in that the mother has experienced labour before and will know what to expect.

The three stages of labour

Labour is divided into three distinct stages.
Stage 1: The onset of regular pains which become stronger and longer, with the interval between each becoming progressively shorter.
Stage 2: The actual birth of the baby.
Stage 3: Delivery of the afterbirth.

STAGE 1

The three signs that labour is starting are a low backache with the onset of regular pains, or 'contractions'; a 'show', seen as a slightly bloodstained mucus stain on the mother's pants; and the 'breaking of the waters'—the amount of fluid lost varies, but the mother's underclothing will be wet. These three signs can occur in any order.

Stage 1 may last for several hours. During the contractions, the birth canal is stretching up to allow the baby through. The Birth Routine continues:

A Use this time to prepare the mother for transfer to hospital. If she is at home, collect her suitcase and hospital documents.
B Take note of how often patient has a contraction and how long it lasts.
C Make sure the mother passes water.
D Reassure her—there is usually plenty of time to get to nospital before the baby arrives.

STAGE 2

But it is occasionally inevitable that the baby is going to arrive first, and the signs of childbirth quickly ensue. The mother will want to bear down and may want to go to the lavatory, or the waters may break, if they have not already done so. Now you must prepare for delivery as follows:

A Find somewhere quiet, private and warm for the mother to lie down (if the mother is in a public place, the need for this should be thought out in advance—during Stage 1).
B Remove tights, pants and underclothes below waist level.
C Collect the following items that you will need:
  —blanket, towel or shawl to keep baby warm (if available kitchen foil may be used it really does retain heat).

118

--blanket to cover the mother.
- -newspapers or plastic sheeting covered with a clean towel or sheet to be placed under mother's bottom.
—swabs or clean handkerchiefs or tissues.
- ·plastic bag.
—sanitary towel or large first aid dressing.

D Wash your hands thoroughly and dry well.

E Assist mother onto her back, ask her to bend her knees and to allow them to fall apart. You will easily see the baby's head when it begins to appear.

F When the mother wants to push or bear down, tell her to hold her breath.

G Place a clean swab over the mother's rectum and wipe away any bowel movement *from the front backwards.*

H Do not interfere as baby's head emerges slowly (Fig. 1). Once the baby's head is delivered, it will turn around—gently support it (Fig. 2).

I The shoulders and body will come out quite quickly. *Do not pull*, but allow the mother to do the pushing (Fig. 3). Be prepared to hold the baby firmly under the armpits. The baby is surprisingly slippery. Lift the baby towards its mother's abdomen.

J Carefully change your grip to hold the baby's ankles and hold baby upside down (Fig. 4). This is to allow any fluid to drain from its mouth and nose, which you should then tidy up with gauze or a handkerchief. The baby will usually cry and breathe regularly at this stage.

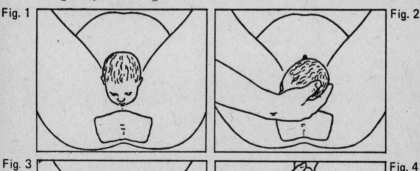

Fig. 1   Fig. 2

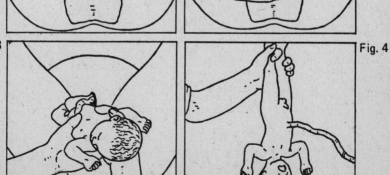

Fig. 3   Fig. 4

119

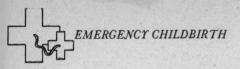

K Remember the child is connected to its mother by the umbilical cord. *Do not pull on the cord.*

L Tell the mother it is a boy or a girl, as the case may be, and that it is normal and well. Wrap the baby up and place it on the mother's abdomen on its front, with the head to one side and wait for Stage 3.

STAGE 3

This stage will take very approximately from ten to twenty minutes. *During this time the cord will lengthen, but do not on any account pull on the cord to speed things up, and do not cut the cord.*

A Just wait for the afterbirth to appear, and when it does, place it in the plastic bag and tuck it in the baby's blanket with the baby. The mother can now have her baby to cuddle.

B Continuing care of the mother is now important. Give her a wash and fix the sanitary towel in position.

C Give the mother a cup of tea (have one yourself!) and encourage her to rest. She will be happier if the room is tidied up.

D Continuing care of the baby is equally important. Make sure the child is warm, and observe it carefully.

E Help of a professional nature may reach you at any time during these procedures, but if there is no sign of it when the mother is tidied up, resting and cuddling her child, telephone to ensure that professional help is coming, and if for any reason it is not, then make alternative arrangements.

Remember that if you are completely cut off from help, for example by snow or flood, you can still get professional advice over the telephone, and this might be necessary should considerable time elapse or any complications develop.

The birth routine

A rapid recapitulation of the birth routine will help to stamp it in your mind.

A Make every effort to obtain professional help.

B Remain calm and unhurried.

C Prepare for mother's comfort and reassure her.

D Collect equipment: blankets for mother and baby, protection for bed, gauze, handkerchiefs and tissues, plastic bag, sanitary towel or large dressing, and handwashing facilities.

E Care during birth: protect baby from injury, clean nose and mouth, hold baby upside down, check baby's breathing, lay baby on mother's abdomen.

F Do not cut cord.

G Await delivery of afterbirth.

H Wrap up baby with afterbirth, and give to mother to cuddle.

I Tidy up mother and equipment.

J Keep baby warm.

Index

Accidents 12–21
  car 97–101
  causes of 14–21
    at work 12
    electricity 14–15
    fires 16
    gas 15
    in sports 12–13
    in the bathroom 18–19
    in the bedroom 19
    in the dining room 18
    in the garage 19
    in the garden shed 19
    in the home 12
    in the kitchen 17–18
    in the sitting room 18
    machinery, power
      driven 16–17
    on the staircase and
      landing 18
    water 15–16, 18–19
  prevention of 14, 16–17
  related to age groups
    110–16
  road 21, 97–101
Adhesives, modern 20
  treatment for 20
    eye 20
    fingers 20
    mouth 20
Adults, injuries 113
Airway
  breathing 33
  clearing 43
Alcohol, unconsciousness
  through 66
  treatment 67
Allergy, acute,
  unconsciousness
  through 67
  treatment 67

Anal bleeding 56
  treatment 56
Anti-coagulants, bleeding
  in casualty on 58
  symptoms 58
  treatment 58
Arm fracture 80
  treatment 80
Arm sling 25–6
  substitutes for 26–7
ARTIFICIAL RESPIRATION
  ROUTINE
  for adults 44–5
  for children 45
  for infants 45
Asthma, acute, failure to
  breathe through
  causes of 46
  treatment 46
Athletics injuries 104

Backbone fracture 78
  treatment 78–9
Back passage, bleeding
  from 56
  treatment 56
Bandage
  conforming 28
  applying 28
  triangular 25–7
  applying 25
  as an arm sling 25–6
  other uses 27
Bat game injuries 103–4
Bathroom and WC 18–19
  accidents in 18–19
  electricity in 19
  hypothermia in 19
Bedroom 19
  accidents in 19
  electric blankets 19

  hot water bottles 19
Birth routine 120
Bites 88–92
  cat 88
    treatment 88
  dog 88
    treatment 88
  octopus 91
  shark 91
  snake 89
    treatment 89
  spider 90
  signs 90
    treatment 90–1
Blankness, short periods
  of 64
Bleeding 50–8
  from the back passage
    56
    treatment 56
  from the liver, spleen or
    kidneys (suspected)
    56–7
  causes of 56
    treatment 58
  from the lungs
    (coughing blood in
    quantity) 54
    treatment 54
  from the nose 53–4
    in older age groups
      53–4
    treatment 53
  from the stomach
    (vomiting blood) 55
    treatment 55
  from the surface 51–3
  from the womb (uterus)
    55
  causes of 55
    treatment 55–6

121

Bleeding (*contd.*)
heavy
procedures 50-1
symptoms of 50
in casualty on anti-
coagulant tablets 58
symptoms of 58
treatment 58
piles (haemorrhoids) 56
treatment 56
unconsciousness through
67
treatment 67
wounds, treatment for
51-3
large 52
torn-off limb 52
with a foreign body in
it 53
with no foreign body in
it 51-2
Blood
coughing from lungs 54
treatment 54
from the back passage
56
treatment 56
from the womb 55
causes 55
treatment 55-6
heavy loss of 50-1
procedures 50-1
symptoms 50
transfusion 50
vomiting from stomach
55
treatment 55
Bones 75-82
dislocations 82
clues 82
treatment 82
fractures 75-82
closed 76
diagnosis of 76-7
open 76-7
treatment
arm 80
backbone (spine) 78-9
chest 80
collar bone 80
face 78
general 77
hand 80
hips 81
limbs, lower 81-2
limbs, upper 80
pelvis 81
shoulder blade 80
special 77-82

Breathing 42-9
artificial respiration
44-5
for children and infants
45
clearing the airway 43
control procedure 49
failure, treatment for
common causes of
45-6
acute asthma 46
choking 46
drowning 45
drugs 46
electric shock 46
gas poisoning 46
lightning 46
suffocation by smoke
45
kiss of life 43-4
for children and infants
44
routines, summary of 49
Burns and scalds 69-74
causes 69
in the elderly 114
in infants 111
treatment(s)
general 70-2
special 72-4
chemical burns 73
chemical splashes in
the eye 73-4
clothes on fire, 72-3
electrical burns 74
rope burn 73
sunburn 73
windburn 73
summary 72

Calamine lotion 24
Car accidents 97-101
Car sports injuries 105
Cardiac compression 46-9
Carving 18
Cat
bite, treatment 88
scratch, treatment 89
Chemical burn 73
treatment 73
Chemical splashes in the
eye 73-4
treatment 73-4
Chest fracture 79
treatment 80
Childbirth, emergency
117-20
assessment of situation
118

birth routine 120
labour 118-20
stage 1 118
stage 2 118-20
stage 3 120
preliminary routine 117
Children, injuries 113
Chilling, cold wet 116
prevention 116
treatment 116
Choking
failure to breathe
through 46
treatment 46
in infants 111
treatment 111
Climbing injuries 107
Closed fracture 76
Clothes on fire 72-3
Cold wet chilling 116
prevention 116
treatment 116
Collar bone fracture 80
in infant 112
treatment 80
Coloured casualty
cyanosis 37
clues 38
shock 37
clues 37
Common accidents 14-
17
Compressed dressings
27-8
applying 27-8
substitutes for 28
Conforming bandages,
applying 28
Consciousness, loss of 33
Continuing care 38-9
Contractions 118
Convulsion,
unconsciousness
through 63
infantile 63
treatment 63
in older child or adult
64
treatment 64
Cookers 17-18
Cooling (hypothermia) in
the elderly 115-16
Coral cut 92
treatment 92
Coronary thrombosis
64-5
treatment 65
Cot or pram, fall from
110

Coughing blood from
  lungs 54
  treatment 54
Cramp 83, 107
  treatment 107
Cuts (minor) 93 5
  dressing 93 5
  renewal of 95
  in infants 93 5, 111
Cyanosis 37-8
Cycle sports injuries 105

D and V, in infants 112
  treatment 112 13
Diabetes, unconsciousness
  through 65
  treatment 65-6
DIAGNOSIS 32
Diarrhoea and vomiting
  in infants 112
  treatment 112-13
Dining room, accidents in
  18
Dislocations 82
  clues 82
  treatment 82
DISPOSAL 30
Dog bite 88
  treatment 88
Dressings
  compressed 27
  applying 27
  substitutes for 28
  minor wounds 93-4
  renewal of 95
Drink, unconsciousness
  through 66
  treatment 67
Drowning 15
  failure to breathe
    through 45
  treatment 45
  unconsciousness through
    68
  treatment 68
Drugs, failure to breathe
  through 46
  treatment 46
Drugs overdose 66
  treatment 66
  conscious casualty 66
  unconscious casualty 66

Ears, infants 110 11
Elderly, common
  accidents in 113-16
  burns 114
  cooling, accidental 115
  fainting 114

fractured limbs 114-15
hip bone fracture (neck
  of femur) 114
heart attack 114
hypothermia 115
  clues 115
  prevention 115
  treatment 116
  nose-bleeds 114
  poisoning 115
  scalds 114
  stroke 114
Electric blankets 19
Electric shock 67-8
  failure to breathe
    through 46
  treatment 46
  unconsciousness through
    67
  treatment 68
Electrical burn 74
  treatment 74
Electricity 14-15
Emergency childbirth
  117 20
Emergency services
  routine 30 1
Epilepsy, unconsciousness
  through 63
EQUIPMENT 22-8
  compressed dressings
    27-8
  applying 27-8
  substitutes for 28
  conforming bandage 28
  applying 28
  first aid box contents
    in the car 24-5
    in the home 23
    for the home 22
  medicine cupboard
    contents 23-4
  triangular bandage 25
    applying 25-7
    as an arm sling 25-7
    other uses of 27
    substitutes for 26-7
EXAMINATION 31-2
Exposure 106
  treatment 106

Face fracture 77
  treatment 78
Failure to breathe
  common causes 45-6
  asthma, acute 46
  choking 46
  drowning 45
  drugs 46

electricity 46
gas poisoning 46
lightning 46
suffocation by smoke
  45
Faint, the common 61
Fainting in the elderly
  114
Fat pan fire 18
Fires 16
First aid box contents
  for the car 24-5
  for the home 23
Fits, minor 64
Football injuries 103
Fracture
  arm 80
    treatment 80
  backbone 78
    treatment 78-9
  chest 79
    treatment 80
  closed 76
  collar bone 80
    treatment 80
  diagnosis of 76-7
  face 77
    treatment 78
  hand 80
    treatment 80
  hip 80-1
    treatment 81
  limbs 80 2
    in the elderly 114 15
    treatment 80, 81-2
  loss of power 76
  open 76 7
  pain 76
  pelvis 80-1
    treatment 81
  shock 76
  shoulder blade
    (suspected) 80
    treatment 80
  skull 77
  spine 78
    treatment 78-9
  swelling 76
  treatment, general
    77
  unusual shape and
    movement 76-7
  wrist 80
    treatment 80
Friction burn 73
  treatment 73
Frostbite 106
  treatment 106
Fuse 14

Gadgets 17
  in the kitchen 17
  in the utility room 17
Game hunting 106
Garage or garden shed 19
  accidents in 19
  inflammable materials in 19
  insecticides in 19
  poisonous materials in 19
  weed killers in 19
Gas 15
  explosive 15
  poisonous 15
Gas poisoning
  failure to breathe through 46
    treatment 46
  unconsciousness through 68
    treatment 68
Grand mal 63
Gymnastics injuries 104

Haemorrhoids (piles) 56
  treatment 56
Hand fracture 80
  treatment 80
Head injury
  in infants 112
  unconsciousness through 62
    clues 62
    treatment 62
Headaches, minor 23–4
Heart attack 64–5
  in the elderly 114
  treatment 65
  unconsciousness through 64–5
HEART MASSAGE ROUTINE 36–7, 46–9
  rates for 36–7
  adults 36, 48
  children 36, 48
  infants 36, 48
Heat exhaustion 109
  clues 109
  treatment 109
Heat stroke 108
  clues 108
  precautions 108
  treatment 108–9
HELP ROUTINE 29–38
  diagnosis 32
  disposal 30
  emergency services 30–1
  examination 31–2

  see, hear and feel 31–2
  shake, shout and pinch 31
  preliminary 29–30
  summary of 38
  treatment 33–7
    priorities 33
    airway 33
    bleeding 33
    consciousness 33
Hip fracture 80–1
  treatment 81
  in the elderly 114
Holiday injuries 102
Horse sports injuries 105
Hot water bottles 19
Hypothermia
  clues 115
  in babies 115
  in other age groups 115
  in the bath 19
  in the elderly 115
  prevention 115
  treatment 116

Infants
  comon accidents in 110–12
  burns 111
  choking 111
    treatment 111
  collar bone (fractured) 112
  cuts 111
  ears 110–11
  falls from cot or pram 110
  head 112
  hypothermia 115
    clues 115
    prevention 115
    treatment 116
  nappy pins 112
  nose 110–11
  poisoning 112
  scalds 111
  suffocation 110
  sunburn 111–12
  sunstroke 111–12
  diarrhoea and vomiting (D and V) 112
    treatment 112–13
Injuries, clues to 31–2
Insect bites and stings 90–1
  in the mouth 90
    treatment 90
  on the skin 90
    treatment 90

Insecticides 19
Insulin 65
Internal bleeding 56–7
  causes of 56
  treatment 58

Jellyfish sting 91
  treatment 91
Joints
  injuries 108
    treatment 108

KISS OF LIFE ROUTINE 34–5, 43–4
  for children and infants 35, 44
Kitchen, accidents in 17 18
Knives 17

Labour 118–20
  stage 1 118
  stage 2 118–20
  stage 3 120
Ligaments, torn 83
Lightning, failure to breathe through 46
  treatment 46
Limbs, fractured 80, 81–2
  treatment 80, 81–2
Lungs, coughing blood from 54
  treatment 54

Machinery, power driven 16–17
Marine creatures, bites and stings 91–2
Medic alert bracelet 29–30, 65
Medicine cupboard contents 23–4
Motor cycle sports injuries 105
Mouth to mouth breathing 34–5
Muscles 83
  sprains 83
    clues 83
    treatment 83
  strains 83
    clues 83
    treatment 83

Nappy pins 112
Nose, infants 110–11
Nose bleeding 53–4
  from high blood pressure 53–4

Nose bleeding (*contd.*)
  in the elderly 114
  in older age groups 53–4
  treatment 53, 54

Octopus bite 91
Open fracture 76–7

Paralysis 78
Pedestrians 21
  precautions 21
Pelvis fracture 80–1
  treatment 81
Pesticides 86–7
Piles (haemorrhoids) 56
  treatment 56
Plant stings 90
 on the skin 90
  treatment 90
Poisons 84–7
 common 85
  treatment, general 86
 in the elderly 115
 in infants 112
 skin 86
  clues 87
  treatment 87
Portuguese man of war
    sting 91
 signs 91
 treatment 91
Pot holing injuries 107
PRIORITIES IN TREATMENT
    33
 airway 33
 bleeding 33
 consciousness 33
Pulled muscle 83
Pulse 39
 feeling 39
 rates for
  adults 39
  children 39
  infants 39

Rabies 88
Racket game injuries
    103–4
RECOVERY POSITION 34
Rectal bleeding 56
 treatment 56
Road accident 21, 97–101
 arriving on the scene
    97–8
 dealing with casualties
    100–101
 information required by
    emergency services
    99

organizing the situation
    98–100
 priorities 98
 safety precautions 99
Rope burn 73
 treatment 73
ROUTINES
 artificial respiration
    44–5
 breathing summary
    49
 emergency services 30–1
 heart massage 36–7,
    46–9
 help 29–38
  continuing care 38–9
  diagnosis 32
  examination 31–2
  priorities 33
  summary of 38
  treatment 33–7
 kiss of life (mouth to
    mouth breathing)
    34–5, 43–4
 recovery position 34
 see, hear and feel 31–2
 shake, shout and pinch
    31
Rugby injuries 103

Sea urchin sting 91–2
 treatment 92
Seat belts 21
See, hear and feel routine
    31–2
Shake, shout and pinch
    routine 31
Shark bite 91
Shell, cone-shaped, sting
    92
 treatment 92
Shock 40
Shoulder blade fracture
    (suspected) 80
 treatment 80
Sitting room, accidents in
    18
Skin, poisoning through
    86
 clues 87
 treatment 87
Skull fracture 77
Sling, arm 25–6
 substitutes for 26–7
Snake bite 89
 treatment 89
Soccer injuries 103
Spider bite 90
 signs 90

treatment 90–1
Spine fracture 78
 paralysis 78
 treatment 78–9
Sports injuries 20,
    102–9
 athletics 104
 big game hunting 106
 climbing 107
 conclusion 109
 conveyance sports 105
 gymnastics 104
 minor 107–8
  cramp 107
   treatment 107
  joints and muscles 108
   treatment 108
  stitch in the side 107
   treatment 107
  winding 107–8
   treatment 107–8
 pot holing 107
 racket, bat and stick
    games 103–4
 rugby 103
 soccer 103
 water sports 104–5
 winter sports 106
Sprains 83
 clues 83
 treatment 83
Staircase and landing,
    accidents on 18
Stick game injuries 103–4
Stings
 cone-shaped shells 92
  treatment 92
 insects 90
  treatment 90
 in the mouth 90
  treatment 90
 jellyfish 91
  treatment 91
 plants 90
  treatment 90
 portuguese man of war
    91
  signs 91
  treatment 91
 sea urchins 91–2
  treatment 92
Stitch in the side 107
 treatment 107
Stomach, vomiting blood
    from 55
 treatment 55
Stoves 17–18
Strains 83
 clues 83

Strains (*contd.*)
  treatment 83
Stroke
  in the elderly 114
  unconsciousness through
    62-3
  clues 62-3
  treatment 63
Suffocation
  by smoke 45
  failure to breathe
    through 45
  treatment 45
  in infants 110
Sunburn 73
  infants 111-12
  treatment 73
Sunstroke, infants 111-12
Swelling around broken
  bones 76

Ticks, treatment 90
Toothache, minor 23-4
Torn ligament 83
TREATMENT 33-7
Triangular bandage
  applying 25-7
  as an arm sling 25-7
  other uses of 27
  substitutes for 26-7

Umbilical cord 120
Unconsciousness 59-68
  causes of 61-8
  allergy, acute 67

treatment 67
bleeding, severe 67
  treatment 67
common faint 61
  treatment 61
convulsion 63
  infantile, treatment 63
  in the older child or
    adult, treatment 64
diabetes 65
  treatment 65-6
drink 66
  treatment 67
drowning 68
  treatment 68
drugs 66
  conscious casualty,
    treatment 66
  unconscious casualty,
    treatment 66
electric shock 67
  treatment 68
epilepsy, convulsions or
  fits 63
fits, minor 64
gas poisoning 68
  treatment 68
head injury 62
  clues 62
  treatment 62
heart attack 64 5
  treatment 65
stroke 62-3
  clues 62-3
  treatment 63

suspected 31
  treatment 59-61

Vomiting and diarrhoea
  in infants 112-13
Vomiting blood from
  stomach 55
  treatment 55

Water
  drowning 15
Water sports injuries
  104-5
Weed killers 19
Wind burn 73
  treatment 73
Winding 107
  treatment 107-8
Winter sports injuries 106
Womb, bleeding from 55
  causes 55
  treatment 55-6
Wound, bleeding 51-3
  treatment 51-3
  with foreign body in it
    53
  without foreign body in
    it 51-2
  large 52
  torn off limbs 52
Wrist fracture 80
  treatment 80

Young people, injuries
  113